stretchfit

STRETCH TO GET FIT AND STAY FIT

KAREN MCCONNELL

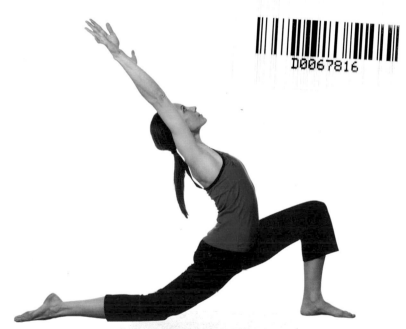

BARRON'S

D0067816

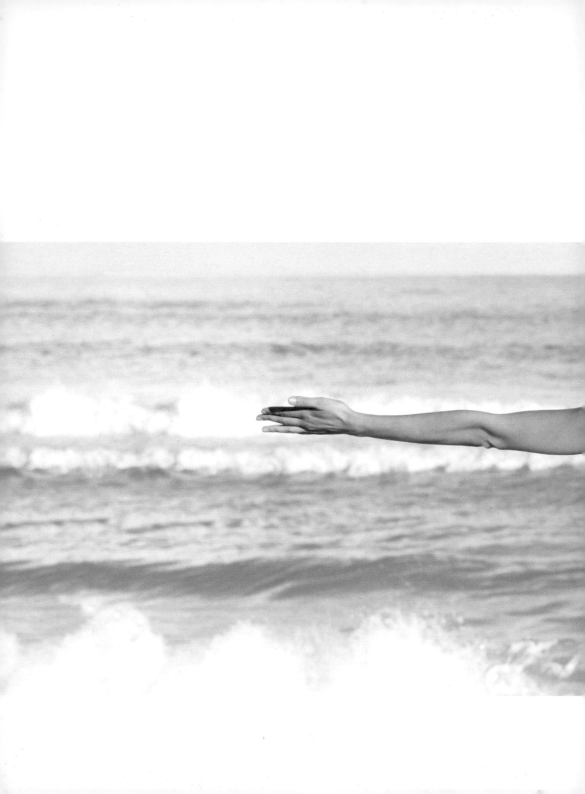

stretchfit

STRETCH TO GET FIT AND STAY FIT

KAREN MCCONNELL

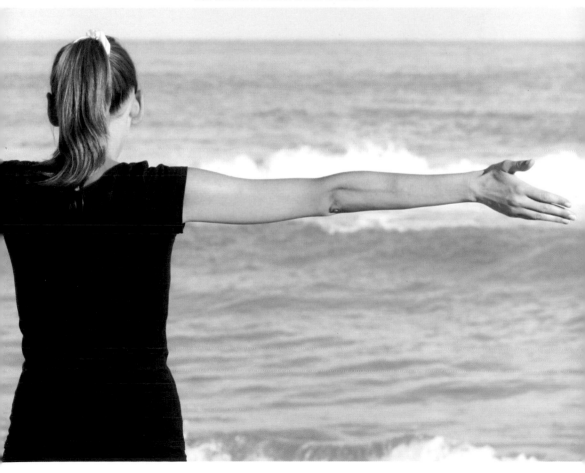

BARRON'S

This edition for the United States, its territories and dependencies, and Canada published in 2011 by Barron's Educational Series, Inc.

Conceived and created by
Axis Publishing Limited
8c Accommodation Road
London NW11 8ED
ww.axispublishing.co.uk

Creative Director: Siân Keogh
Designer: Sean Keogh
Project Editor: Anna Southgate
Production: Bili Books

NOTE
The opinions and advice expressed in this book are intended as a guide only. The publisher and author accept no responsibility for any injury or loss sustained as a result of using this book.

All inquiries should be addressed to:
Barron's Educational Series, Inc.
250 Wireless Blvd.
Hauppauge, NY 11788
www.barronseduc.com

Library of Congress Control Number:
2011926819

ISBN 13: 978-0-7641-4687-9

Printed in China
9 8 7 6 5 4 3 2 1

contents

foreword   6

introduction   8

benefits of flexibility   10

active or passive stretching   12

the daily stretch   14

aerobic fitness   16

great aerobic workouts   18

measuring your heart rate   20

nutrition and hydration   22

core strength and stability   26

lower body stretches   28

stretches 1–3   30

stretches 4–7   32

stretches 8–11   34

stretches 12–15   36

stretches 16–20   38

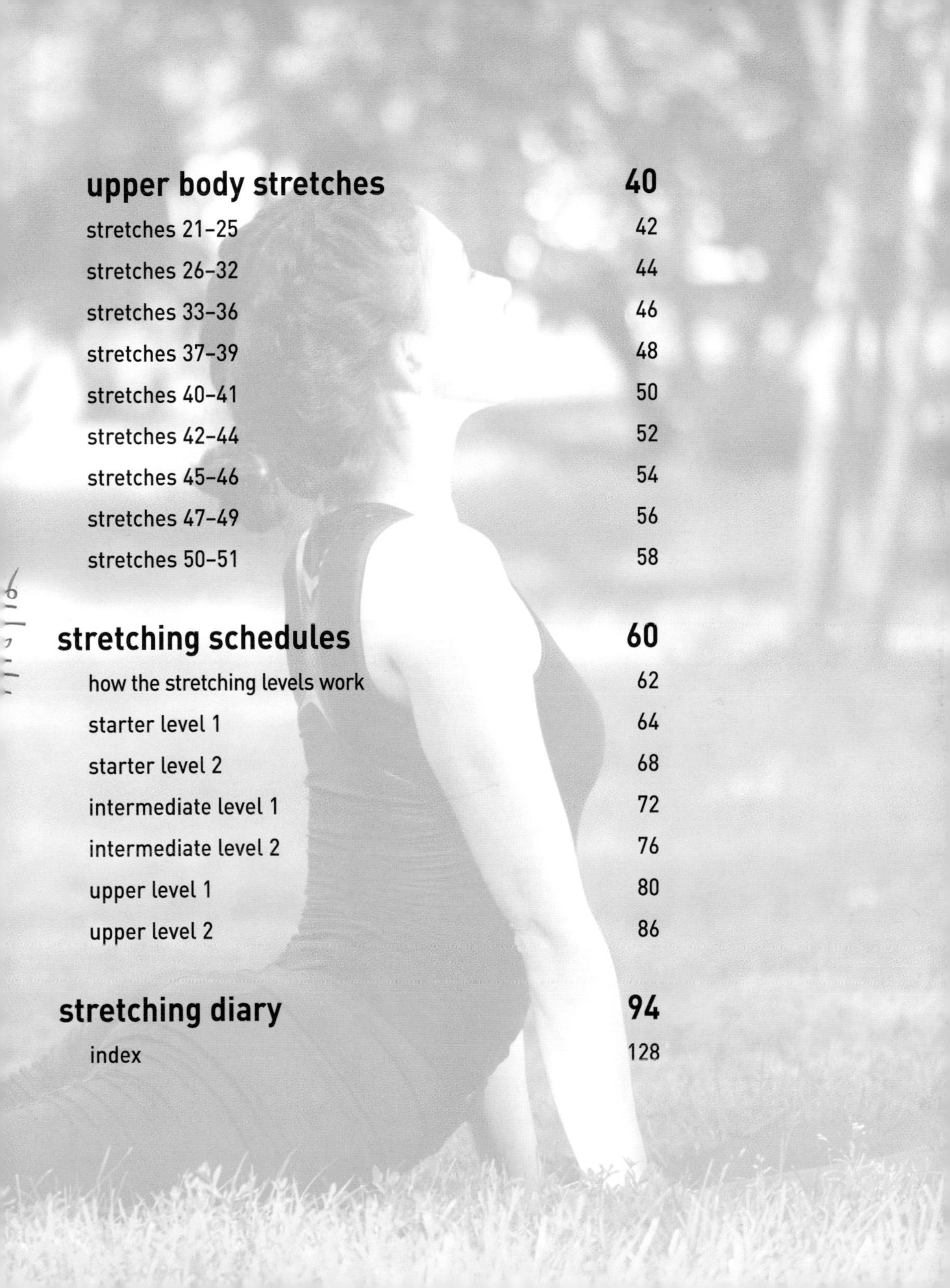

upper body stretches   **40**

stretches 21–25   42

stretches 26–32   44

stretches 33–36   46

stretches 37–39   48

stretches 40–41   50

stretches 42–44   52

stretches 45–46   54

stretches 47–49   56

stretches 50–51   58

stretching schedules   **60**

how the stretching levels work   62

starter level 1   64

starter level 2   68

intermediate level 1   72

intermediate level 2   76

upper level 1   80

upper level 2   86

stretching diary   **94**

index   128

foreword

I still remember the first article on stretching that I ever read: It was the mid-1980s and it was an article published in *Runner's World* magazine promoting the benefits of this new training technique called stretching. At the time I was an enthusiastic young athlete, competing in track and triathlon, and I was willing to give anything a go in the hope of improving my personal best times.

That was the beginning of a journey for me that I am still on today. From that day forward I started looking for more information on stretching and flexibility training, and I started to apply some of the techniques I was learning.

Back in the 1980s you could barely find a one-page article on stretching with a few images of stick figures in it. Today, there are dozens of books on the topic, and slowly but surely more and more people are recognizing the benefits of stretching for improved range of motion and better posture, for developing body awareness, improving coordination, and for simple relaxation and stress relief.

If you've never tried stretching before, you owe it to yourself to give it a go. A regular stretching program, like the routines outlined in this book, will help you enhance your athletic ability, decrease the likelihood of sports injury, and minimize muscle soreness.

If nutrition is important to you, then stretching should be too. If cardiovascular fitness and strength training are a priority for you, then so is stretching.

Don't make the mistake of thinking that something as simple as stretching won't be effective. Add some simple stretching exercises to your fitness program today.

Brad Walker
Founder & CEO
The Stretching Institute™

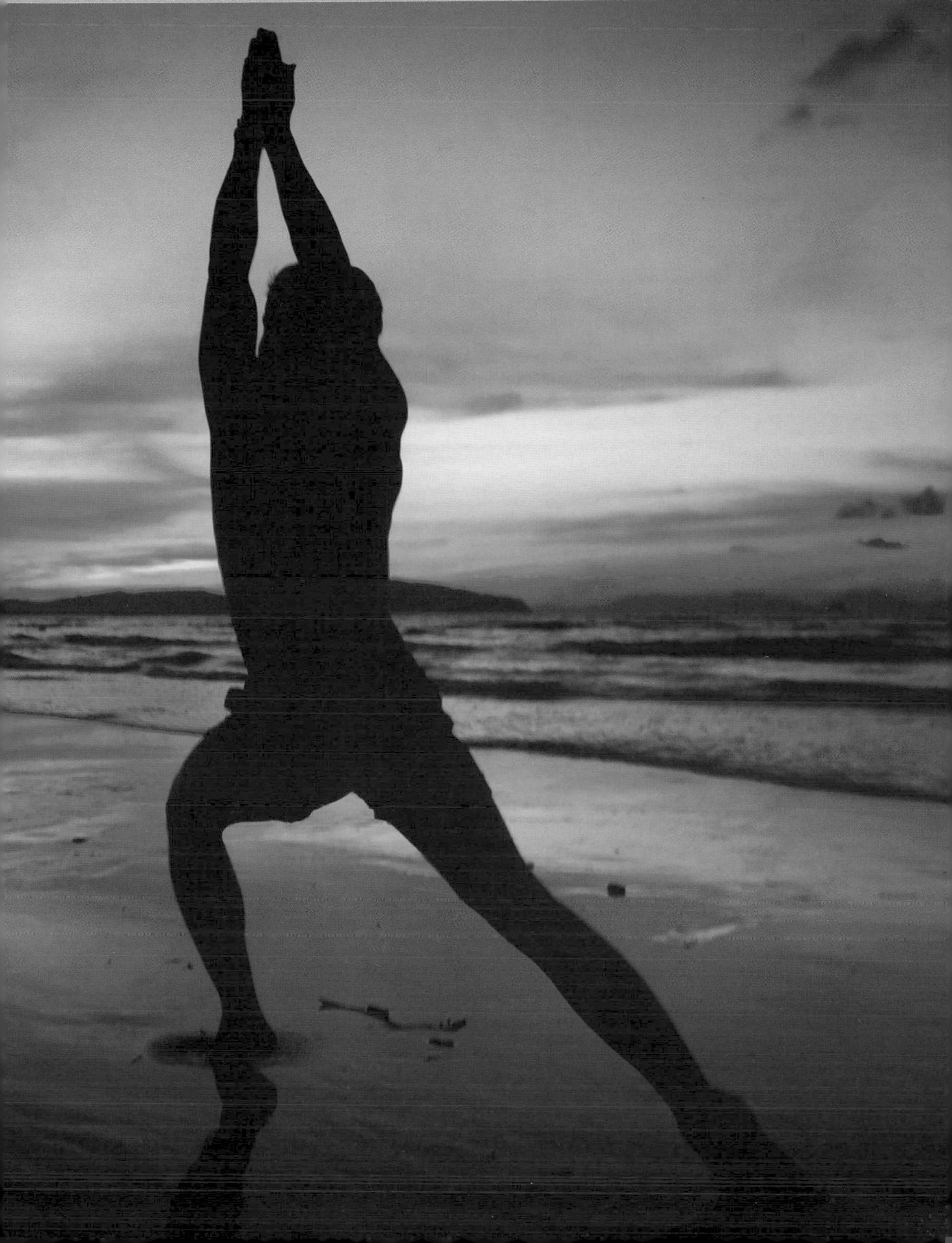

introduction

Welcome to Stretchfit. The schedules in this book are designed to help you get fit and flexible safely and effectively, and whether you are a complete beginner or a serious athlete there are schedules to help you achieve your fitness goals. Using the stretching programs will also help to address all those built-up postural imbalances that result in some muscles and joints being tight, while others are relatively weak or loose.

As a start to your return to fitness this stretching regime will get you in touch with your body and help you to understand how it works as a series of interconnected and interdependent parts. Stretching will help to prepare your muscles and joints for increasing your levels of activity and reduce the risk of injuries that can strike just when you begin to feel you are achieving your goals.

Stretching should not be painful! Go as far into any stretch as far as you can comfortably and then, with the aid of deep breathing, allow the muscles to release. Some of the deeper muscles can take up to a minute to begin to change so don't be in a hurry.

Doing smaller amounts on a regular basis will be more effective than one big session a week. Little and often! Ten minutes of stretching every day will make a big difference with 2 to 3 longer sessions per week to progress things along.

Some of the progressions are very strong stretches; if you find you are very achy after a stretch session, it may be that you are not ready for that particular intensity yet, so go back to the previous version you were comfortable with for a week or two and then try it again.

Strengthening should be part of any exercise regime as building muscle size and muscle tone helps to support and protect the joints. You don't have to be a bodybuilder! Many of the stretches in the latter parts of the schedules involve body weight exercises such as push ups and squats. Don't worry if you have not done one in years or if you never have. You can start by using the weight of your arms and legs;

raising your outstretched arms above your head; and straightening and bending your knees while you are sitting down. Some of the exercises are weight based and a target number of repetitions is given. If you can't complete the given number, do as much as you can and repeat that number over the next few sessions until you feel comfortable; then increase by 10% or no more than 30%. Repeat again until comfortable and increase again by no more than 30%. If you cannot complete the action at all, try a less vigorous version just using the weight of that part of your body, or taking the movement less far.

To progress from body weight you can use small household objects such as a bottle of water or a small can of food to strengthen your arm and shoulder muscles; holding a larger juice carton will work your legs, back, and abdominals when doing squats and lunges.

With the strength work increase the number of repetitions so that you do 2 sets of 5–10 reps and then add on repetitions so that as you get to the end of the second set you have to work quite hard to complete it. With the standing strength exercises it is very important to maintain good posture throughout. If by the end of the second set you cannot hold the position, you are probably doing too many reps. It's not just about the weight!

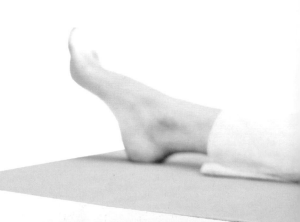

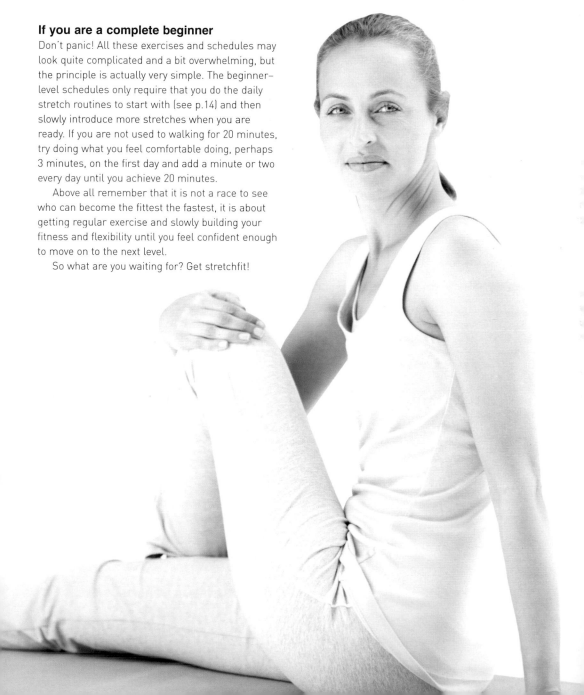

If you are a complete beginner

Don't panic! All these exercises and schedules may look quite complicated and a bit overwhelming, but the principle is actually very simple. The beginner–level schedules only require that you do the daily stretch routines to start with (see p.14) and then slowly introduce more stretches when you are ready. If you are not used to walking for 20 minutes, try doing what you feel comfortable doing, perhaps 3 minutes, on the first day and add a minute or two every day until you achieve 20 minutes.

Above all remember that it is not a race to see who can become the fittest the fastest, it is about getting regular exercise and slowly building your fitness and flexibility until you feel confident enough to move on to the next level.

So what are you waiting for? Get stretchfit!

benefits of flexibility

This book is designed to provide an understanding of flexibility so that the reader can achieve a healthy flexibility that will improve his or her posture, fitness, and general well-being.

Everyone should perform stretching exercises, whether or not they use it as a preparation for sports and other activities. Many people who do regular exercise tend to focus on their fitness, strength, and endurance and spend very little time improving their flexibility. Flexibility is one of the essential components of fitness because it improves performance and reduces muscular tension. An absence of stretching has been shown to increase the potential for injury through tight or stiff muscle fibers and create closed, unhealthy postures.

Flexibility is specific to individual joints and the ability of those joints to move through their full range of movement (ROM) with little resistance from the surrounding muscle tissue. ROM varies from one joint to the next and according to the kind of activity performed. Everyday living requires a certain ROM for healthy flexibility, whereas specific physical activities may need the ROM of particular joints to be much more flexible.

static and dynamic training

There are two main types of flexibility training: static, which is when a muscle is held stretched for a length of time; and dynamic, which involves slow or fast movement into stretched positions that are not held. Static flexibility training concentrates on individual muscles and joints whereas dynamic training uses multiple muscles and joints combined with neuromuscular coordination and strength. Dynamic movements are important because they are specific to everyday activity, but they risk a greater chance of injury due to the speed and force of the stretch.

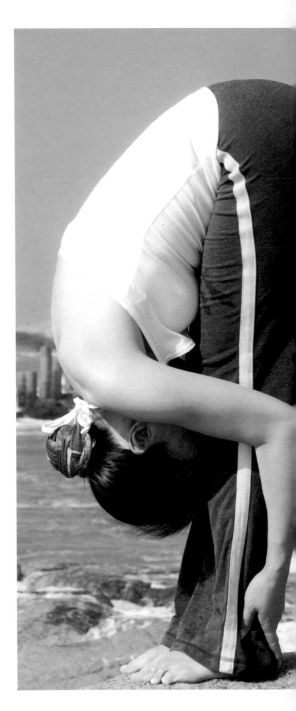

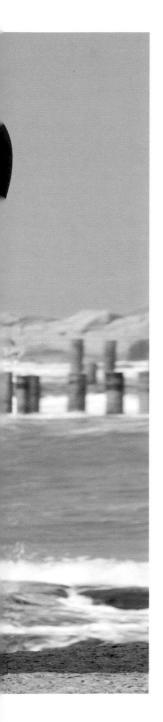

IMPROVED MOVEMENT

Flexibility can improve physical performance. As there is less tissue resistance, it requires less energy to achieve the ROM. With less tissue resistance there is a decreased chance of injury as you are less likely to exceed the tissue's extensibility during movements.

INCREASED BLOOD SUPPLY

By moving joints through the full ROM, there is an increase in blood and nutrient supply to the joint structures, improving health and mobility. Greater ROM exercise increases the quantity of synovial fluid (the protective lubricant that aids joint movement) and increases the viscosity of the fluid to allow greater and easier movement with more efficient nutrient transportation. An increase in synovial fluid may reduce the degeneration of joint structures, which can cause arthritic conditions.

BETTER MUSCLE COORDINATION

Flexibility improves neuromuscular coordination. The time taken for messages to travel from the muscle to the brain is reduced due to the adaptation of the nervous tissue and its ability to isolate muscle response.

IMPROVED POSTURE AND BALANCE

Flexibility training encourages better resting muscle tension to improve postural balance and awareness. It helps realign soft tissue structures that may have adapted to closed postural positions. Realignment reduces the effort needed to adopt good posture.

RELIEVES LOWER BACK PAIN

Lower back pain can be reduced by an increase in lumbar and pelvic movement, which is improved by elongating the hamstrings, hip flexors, gluteals, and lumbar muscles.

RELIEVES MUSCLE STRESS

Stretching is an excellent method of relieving muscular stress and mental tension. Tense muscles have reduced blood supply. They also have a greater toxicity that may cause lethargy. Better muscle equilibrium creates a sense of vitality and well-being.

active or passive stretching

Active stretching is the contraction of the antagonistic muscle to provide force against the stretched muscle. For example, when the leg is raised straight in front of the body, the quadriceps (at the front of the thigh) contract while the hamstrings (at the back of the thigh) become stretched. Active stretching strengthens the contracting muscles and reduces the stretch resistance of the elongated muscles. Active stretching is better with the dynamic technique, although it does not lead to as much muscle development as the passive method. However, the combined use of strength with coordination is more common among athletes, who develop muscles for particular activities.

Passive stretching is when the muscle being stretched has an external force applied to it. For example, in an upright hamstring stretch, where the resting foot is place on an object of knee height or

OVERCOMING LIMITED FLEXIBILITY

Some people, especially beginners, may not have the flexibility to perform some stretches in their entirety. If this is the case, a towel can be a very useful aid to gaining a full and effective stretch.

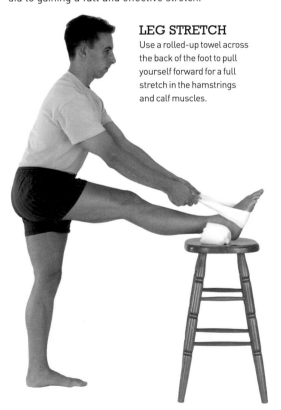

LEG STRETCH
Use a rolled-up towel across the back of the foot to pull yourself forward for a full stretch in the hamstrings and calf muscles.

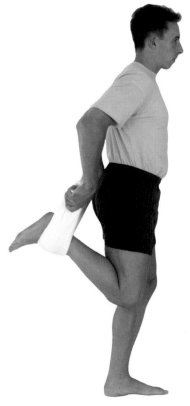

above, the force applied is the weight of the body leaning over the stretched leg. This does not require voluntary contractions in any of the muscles.

Sometimes it is better to stretch to gain both plastic (static/passive) and elastic (dynamic/active) elongation. For example, a martial arts expert is able to kick very high, the height of the kick being determined by the strength in the quadriceps and the stretch resistance in the hamstrings. If the expert were to use the static technique of stretching to achieve permanent elongation, the kick would become much higher with less risk of injury due to an increase in the tissue's extensibility. This would require less force from the working muscles. If the static technique were combined with the dynamic technique,

a greater amount of strength and coordination would achieve a higher kick with less effort.

For good health we do not need this amount of ROM, but should have a good static flexibility. Beginners should aim for plastic elongation through static stretching until optimum movement is achieved. Only after having achieved the best you can from static movement is it advisable to improve dynamic flexibility.

tissue damage

When plastic elongation occurs there is some tissue damage, which can cause mild muscle soreness. The weakness is only short term while molecular reconstruction creates a new resting length for the muscle. For example, if we take a hot steel rod and pull both ends until it lengthens, the metal becomes weak at the point of elongation due to the molecular reconstruction. As the metal cools the strength is regained. Overstretching can lead to serious tissue damage and reduce flexibility. Another factor affecting elongation is temperature. When body temperature increases by just a few degrees, there is a reduced muscle resistance and greater muscle elasticity. A high-force, short-duration stretch at normal or above average temperatures will induce elastic elongation and a temporary gain in flexibility. Alternatively, a low-force, long duration stretch at high temperatures will produce long-term plastic deformation.

QUADRICEPS STRETCH

If you cannot reach your ankle with your hand, use a rolled-up towel to pull your foot up to gain a stretch in the front of the thigh.

HAMSTRINGS STRETCH

A towel can help raise the leg up to a 90-degree angle to gain a stretch along the back of the leg. This static style of stretching will help achieve plastic elongation of the muscle.

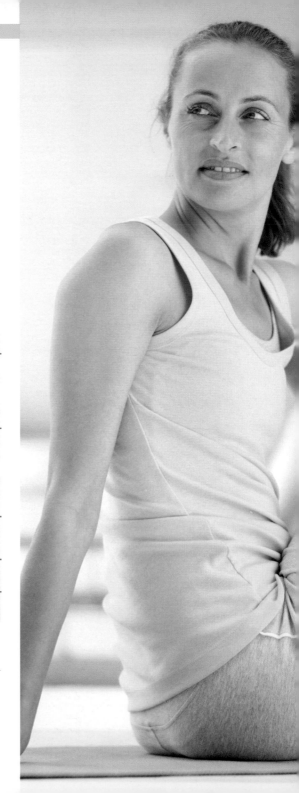

the daily stretch

The daily stretch is just that, whether you are working out or not, and even on rest days, you should do these daily stretch routines, and the 20-minute daily walk.

LEVELS 1–3 (see pages 64–75)

WEEK 1 and every day throughout the schedule. This should take no more than 10 minutes.

LYING FACE UP

1	single knee hugs (p 35)
2	feet down knee rotation (p 38)

LYING FACE DOWN

3	quad stretch (p 36)
4	sphinx (p 44)

SITTING / STANDING

5	raise straight arms in front and then above head 5x with breath (p 42–43)
6	raise straight arms to side and then above head 5x with breath (p 42–43)
7	neck simple rotation (p 43)
8	standing neck stretch (p 43)

20-minute daily walk.

Generally increase levels of activity; walking up and down stairs and escalators, getting off the bus or train a stop or two before your destination, walking a little faster, making local journeys on your bicycle, or visiting the local swimming pool.

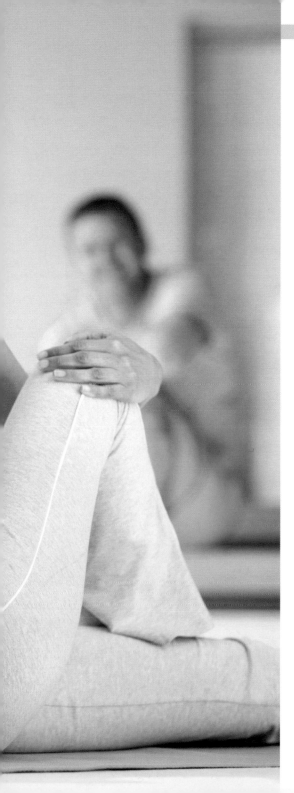

LEVELS 4–6 (see pages 76–93)

WEEK 1 and every day throughout the schedule. This should take no more than 15 minutes.

LYING FACE UP

| 1 | single knee hugs (p 35) |
| 2 | feet down knee rotation (p 38) |

LYING FACE DOWN

3	quad stretch (p 36)
4	sphinx (p 44)
5	Cat into Cow 5x each with fingers forward, pointing in, pointing out (p 47)

LYING ON YOUR SIDE

| 6 | chalk circles (p 46) |

SITTING / STANDING

7	raise straight arms in front and then above head 5x with breath (p 42-43)
8	raise straight arms to side and then above head 5x with breath (p 42-43)
9	neck simple rotation (p 43)
10	standing neck stretch (p 43)

20-minute daily walk.

Generally increase levels of activity; walking up and down stairs and escalators, not parking as close as possible to your destination, walking a little faster, and checking the road worthiness of your old bicycle and the opening times of your local swimming pool.

aerobic fitness

Developing and maintaining good heart and lung function delivers aerobic fitness, which itself is one of the main cornerstones of any workout program.

Exercise programs need to contain three essential ingredients: aerobic exercise, training for muscular strength, and promoting flexibility. The first of these, aerobic exercise, improves your cardiovascular (CV) fitness—the strength and efficiency of your heart and lungs—as well as toning the rest of the muscles in your body. Aerobic exercise is any activity that uses large muscle groups over an extended period of time. It is called aerobic fitness because it involves taking in, transporting, and using oxygen in your muscles. Your fitness improves as the efficiency of this process improves—a process that is driven by your heart and lungs.

WHEN BEST TO EXERCISE

Our bodies respond to exercise better at some points during the day than at others. The body's natural cycles are called circadian rhythms and these control our body temperature. During the day, our body temperature changes, peaking in the late afternoon, and falling to its lowest point in the small hours of the morning. Generally, our bodies work best when their temperatures are high—our muscles are warmer and more relaxed, perceived exertion is low, and reaction times are quicker. We are stronger and our resting heart rates are lower. However, if you are aiming to train for a specific event, such as a 10 k running race, a half-marathon, or even a marathon that has an early morning start, it is better to train in the early morning. It seems that you can adapt your circadian rhythms to deliver the best performance when you need it most.

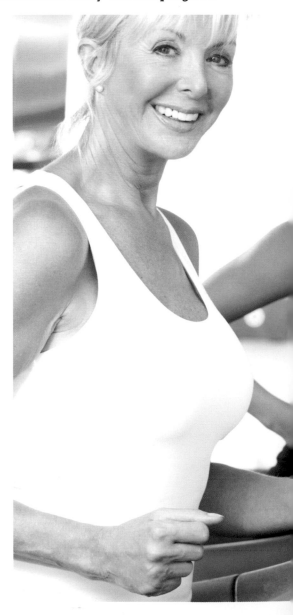

HOW TO IMPROVE YOUR CV FITNESS

Any activity that raises your heart rate and leaves you even moderately out of breath will improve your CV fitness. These include favorites such as jogging, cycling, and swimming, but dance classes or brisk walking also work. Here are some tips:

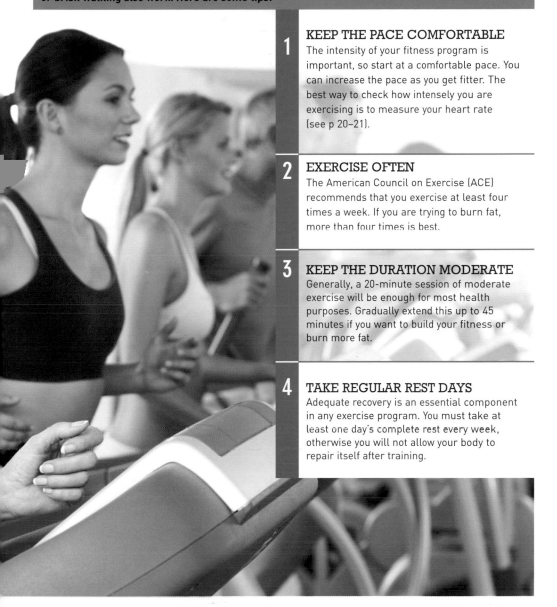

1 KEEP THE PACE COMFORTABLE

The intensity of your fitness program is important, so start at a comfortable pace. You can increase the pace as you get fitter. The best way to check how intensely you are exercising is to measure your heart rate (see p 20–21).

2 EXERCISE OFTEN

The American Council on Exercise (ACE) recommends that you exercise at least four times a week. If you are trying to burn fat, more than four times is best.

3 KEEP THE DURATION MODERATE

Generally, a 20-minute session of moderate exercise will be enough for most health purposes. Gradually extend this up to 45 minutes if you want to build your fitness or burn more fat.

4 TAKE REGULAR REST DAYS

Adequate recovery is an essential component in any exercise program. You must take at least one day's complete rest every week, otherwise you will not allow your body to repair itself after training.

great aerobic workouts

So which workouts provide aerobic fitness? Below is just a sample of the myriad of different exercises you can do outdoors, in the gym, in the pool, and in classes.

We've already noted that any exercise that raises your pulse for more than about 20 minutes will improve fitness, but what about if you really want to improve your aerobic fitness? Here are some ideas:

running

All you need is some good-quality running shoes, clothing that is appropriate to the climate, and some open sidewalks. As well as a great CV workout, running strengthens your legs and is a great fat burner and stress buster—there's nothing like getting moving in the great outdoors to clear your head.

treadmill

If the weather is terrible or the streets are just too crowded or polluted, there's always the treadmill at the gym. This requires its own technique, since you are running on a moving belt. Relax into it, keeping your head up.

bicycle

Just like running, getting out in the open air is a cathartic experience, and cycling is a fantastic workout, strengthening your legs and burning fat. Whole exercise and race programs can be developed around this sport. Just be careful of the traffic.

stationary bike

If the weather is too bad, or the traffic is too threatening, the stationary bike is a great alternative and is very versatile. Adjust the seat properly so as not to put too much pressure on your back or knees. Go to some spinning classes for a high-intensity workout that will leave you invigorated.

stairclimber

Another gym favorite, this strengthens the legs, especially the muscles on the front of the thighs (the quadriceps). Make sure you don't push the stair all the way down, or let it come all the way up—this aggravates your knees and back.

rowing machine

Short of belonging to a rowing club (and getting out on the water is a wonderful experience), the next best thing is the rowing machine. Make sure you adjust the difficulty level to suit you, and row in this order: legs-body-arms. Don't pull with your back. Rowing strengthens your legs, chest, and arms.

skier

Not the easiest to use, but a fantastic workout for your gluteus maximus (your butt) and your quadriceps, depending on how you use it. Get used to the rhythm of the machine and the leg and arm movements involved before trying to pick up the pace.

swimming

One of the best all-over body workouts you can get, swimming exercises almost every major muscle group in the body, especially if you try all the swim strokes. It all takes place in the low-impact, supportive environment of water.

boxing, boxercise, and martial arts

These are high-impact, high-intensity activities that test your fitness. They promote all-over body strength, flexibility, balance, and coordination. You may have to attend a class to do these activities, which is motivating, fun, and sociable.

aerobics

Similar to above, and a real fat burner. Again, done in a group or class, you will be motivated to work hard and have fun. There are classes for people at all levels of fitness.

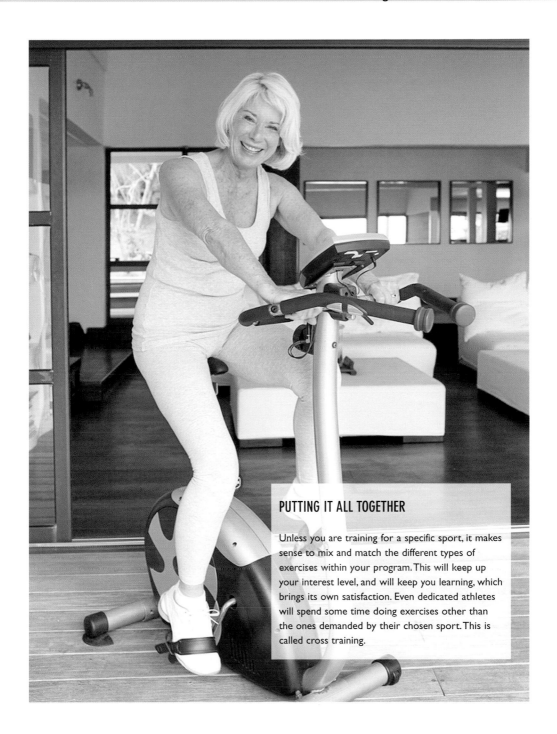

PUTTING IT ALL TOGETHER

Unless you are training for a specific sport, it makes sense to mix and match the different types of exercises within your program. This will keep up your interest level, and will keep you learning, which brings its own satisfaction. Even dedicated athletes will spend some time doing exercises other than the ones demanded by their chosen sport. This is called cross training.

measuring your heart rate

Calculating and planning the intensity of a workout is just as important as simply timing its duration—you need to know how hard to work, as well as how long.

Measuring the intensity of your workouts is important to get the most from your efforts. This applies as much to beginners, who need to make sure they are starting out at a comfortable pace, as it does to more experienced athletes, who need to tailor-make their training so as to maximize the benefits of each session.

monitoring the heart

A heart rate monitor is the easiest way to measure your heart rate, which is calculated in beats per minute (bpm). These monitors consist of a strap that fits around your chest, over your heart, and a watch-type display to which information from the working heart is relayed.

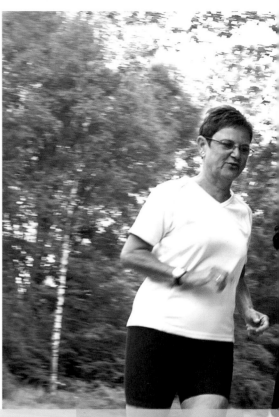

DOING THE MATH

Your training sessions should be based around percentages of what is known as your "working" heart rate.

This is how to calculate it:

Work out your maximum heart rate
To do this, use this formula:

men: 214 – (0.8 x age)

women: 209 – (0.9 x age)

So for example, a 30-year-old woman will have a maximum heart rate of:

209 – (0.9 x 30) = 182

Work out resting heart rate

To do this, take your pulse when you have just woken up in the morning. Take the number of beats you can feel in your wrist over a 15-second period, then multiply by four.
So for example, the same woman may have counted 14 beats over a 15-second period.

14 x 4 = 56

INTENSITY AS PERCENTAGES

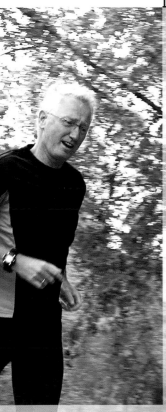

Your target heart rates will of course change depending on the intensity you want to work out at. These are the percentages that are commonly used, and what they mean.

60 percent
Easy. This is an easy session or a recovery session, and is very slow. Sustainable over long periods, up to around three hours.

60–70 percent
Easy. This is a slightly faster pace. At around 65 percent, your body is learning to use fat as fuel. Sustainable over long periods, up to around three hours.

70–85 percent
Moderate. A moderate pace with fast, explosive bursts (in running, this is called "fartlek" training). Sustainable over moderate periods, for example, up to 45 minutes.

90+ percent
Hard. A fast pace, up to peak heart rate. Often used in "interval training," where high heart rates are held for short periods of time, say one minute, before falling to around 70 percent, then increased again, then falling back. Sustainable for short periods of time.

Subtract your resting heart rate from your maximum heart rate

182 – 56 = 126

So 126 is your working heart rate. This is the figure to use, rather than your maximum heart rate.

The final step
Last, use this number to calculate your "target" heart rate. Your target heart rate is based on percentages of your working heart rate, to which you add your resting heart rate.

So if the 30-year-old woman is doing an easy workout, say at 60 percent of her working heart rate, her target heart rate for that session is:

(126 x 60%) + 56 = 132

132 is the number she will want to see on her heart rate monitor for the duration of her workout.

nutrition and hydration

Fueling your body properly will not only help you to realize the full benefits of your exercise program, but also to live a healthier, more energized life.

Part of any exercise program is proper nutrition. This means taking in the right balance of carbohydrates, proteins, fats, vitamins and minerals, and water. These elements provide the fuel that will help you maximize your potential during your workouts, recover during your rest days, and boost your long-term health, minimizing the risks associated with high-fat, nutritionally poor diets, such as heart disease and even some types of cancer. These are the food groups you should be aiming to eat:

carbohydrates ("carbs")

These are the main energy providers. They are divided into two groups: simple carbs and complex carbs. Simple carbs include sugars found in fruit and sports drinks; complex carbs are found in starch-based foods, such as potatoes, rice, and pasta. You will need both in your diet and both are absorbed by the body at different speeds.

Generally, simple carbs tend to provide an immediate source of energy, since they are absorbed very quickly by the body. Complex carbs tend to be absorbed more slowly and provide more sustained energy release. The actual speed at which carbs are absorbed is measured by the Glycemic Index (GI).

Eat carbohydrates before a training session for energy, and after training to replenish your energy levels. As a general guide, you should aim to get around 55 percent of your daily calorie intake from carbs.

Aim to get 55 percent of your daily calories from carbohydrates.

HOW MUCH SHOULD I EAT?

You can calculate how much food you should eat using this formula as a good starting point. Be aware though, that it is only a guide—all bodies are different. Do this math:

METABOLIC RATE		LIFESTYLE		EXERCISE		SO FOR EXAMPLE:
Work out your basal metabolic rate, this is determined by your gender.		**Add 30–40 percent if you have a sedentary job (e.g. office work).**		**Add approximately 400 calories per hour of training.**		A 165 lb (75 kg) male bicycle courier who works out for one hour per day needs:
men: 11 calories per lb of body weight (24 calories per kg)	**+**		**+**		**=**	**165 x 11 = 1,815 + (60% x 1,815) = 2,904 + 400**
		Add 50–60 percent if you have an active job (e.g. construction work).				
women: 10 calories per lb of body weight (22 calories per kg)						**= 3,304 calories**

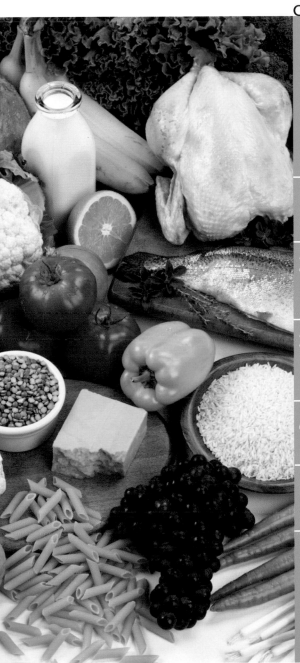

CONTROLLING YOUR WEIGHT

"Losing weight" can be a misleading term. Even if you lose fat through exercise, the extra muscle you build can outweigh the fat you've burned off. Despite this, be aware that weight loss and fat loss are often commonly used to mean the same thing.

To shed that fat try these steps:

1 Take a look at what you eat and see where the bad influences are. Replace these with some healthier alternatives.

2 Take small steps. Don't attempt to alter your eating habits straight away—you may find the change too difficult to stick to.

3 Don't expect too much too soon. Weight loss is a long-term project; despite what the diet industry will tell you, there are no quick fixes.

4 Eat small amounts often. Small healthy snacks are used up more quickly by the body than a few big meals.

5 Exercise more. Every minute spent exercising and not spent sedentary is calories burned. It all adds up.

6 Aim to burn 500 calories a day more than you eat. This will allow you to gradually and safely shed fat. Diets that encourage you to lose 1,000 calories or more a day do not work well because your body goes into starvation mode and actually tries to retain as much weight as possible.

nutrition and hydration continued

protein

Protein provides the building blocks for growth and post-workout muscle repair. Without it, your muscles cannot recover from exercise. Good sources of protein include meat, fish, and poultry, but dairy products, beans, grains, and nuts are also useful. Aim to get about 15 percent of your calories from protein, with a small amount at every meal. Excess protein is simply stored as fat—you don't need the large amounts training manuals often prescribe.
Aim to get 15 percent of your daily calories from protein.

fats

Fats get bad press, but they are a good source of energy, provide protective layering around internal organs, and carry fat-soluble vitamins. Saturated fats, such as those found in dairy products and red meat, are high in cholesterol, which clogs your arteries and can lead to high blood pressure and heart problems. These should be minimized. By contrast, mono- and polyunsaturated fats, such as those found in oily fish, nuts, and olive oil, are healthier. Make them around 30 percent of your daily calorie intake.
Aim to get 30 percent of your daily calories from healthy fats.

vitamins and minerals

Vitamins are organic compounds that help regulate carbohydrate, protein, and fat metabolism in the body. They play a vital role in releasing the energy stored in the foods we eat. In addition, they regulate our nervous, hormonal, and immune systems. Minerals are inorganic elements that have many roles including the formation of strong bones and teeth, control of the nervous system, and regulation of fluid balance and muscle activity. Both vitamins and minerals are essential for good health and growth. Eating plenty of fresh fruit and vegetables should provide you with all the vitamins and minerals you need, although supplements are also available to meet any shortfall.

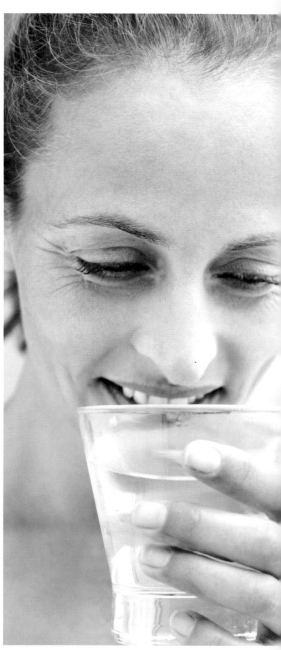

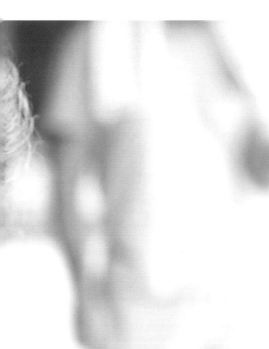

hydration

Part of fueling your body for exercise is drinking plenty of water. In fact, your body will shut down very quickly if it becomes too dehydrated. Most of us do not drink enough water in everyday life, which can leave us feeling lethargic and struggling to stay alert. In terms of following an exercise program, dehydration is a major factor in poor athletic performance. Bear in mind that your body can lose up to 4 pints (2 liters) of water when exercising outdoors on a hot day. In fact, your body needs to take in twice as much water as it loses through sweat in order to restore its proper fluid balance.

what should I drink?

Water is the obvious choice, and for most general purposes, the best. However, sports drinks, fruit juice, and milk are all good as well—just be careful of their calorie content (water has no calories). Try to avoid caffeinated drinks such as tea, coffee, and cola, as well as alcohol. These have "diuretic" properties, meaning that they stimulate the flow of urine, which contributes to dehydration.

HERE'S HOW TO STAY HYDRATED

1 On a nontraining day, drink around eight glasses of water a day.

2 On a training day, look to add at least an extra 50 percent to this total, making around 12 glasses a day.

3 Drink water with every meal.

4 Carry a bottle with you when in the car or on the plane and sip it. Air conditioning and heating systems are very dehydrating.

5 To accurately work out how much water you need, do this math:

½ fl oz per lb (25 ml per kg) of body weight + 34 fl oz (1 l) per hour of exercise.

For example, a 120 lb (55 kg) person will need:
2½ pints (1.4 l) on a nontraining day
4 pints (2.4 l) on a training day, where there is one hour of exercise.

core strength and stability

Core strength and stability training have become an integral part of all fitness regimes as evidence has built up about how such exercises affect the way we use our bodies and protect our lower backs.

Many people taking up or returning to exercise will find themselves experiencing more back pain than before but DON'T GIVE UP. Give some time to learn these techniques and they will help you to get the most out of stretching for fitness.

Where are the core muscles?

The transversus abdominus lies between the bony prominences on the front of the hip bones (ASIS) and its job is to pull in the lower part of the abdomen (between the umbilicus and the pubic bone) as if you were trying to zip up a tight pair of pants.

The pelvic floor muscles are internal muscles in the triangle between the pubic bone at the front and the sitting bones (ischeal tuberosities) at the back, which you would use to stop yourself passing water. The action of these muscles is to internally pull upward from underneath. If you are not sure, try to stop your urine mid-flow by contracting the muscles and release them again.

By learning to consciously control these muscles you will also activate small muscles around the lumbar spine, forming an internal, protective corset.

EXERCISE 1

Lie flat on your back on the floor or on a firm bed with a comfortable curve in your lower back.

Place your fingertips on the abdomen just in from the front ridge of the hip bones (ASIS). Breathe in and as you breathe out pull the lower tummy muscles in toward the spine, and pull the pelvic floor muscles up. The fingertips should feel a tightening of the abdominal muscles, not pushing out. Also, the buttock muscles (glutei) should not contract and the pelvis should not tip or tilt. It's all internal!

Once you feel you can contract the correct muscles the exercise is to lie flat as above and repeat the contractions as you breathe out for 10 seconds at a time, 10 times, once a day, making a "hundred."

EXERCISE 2

Now that you can identify and use your core muscles you must become used to using them in normal daily activities.

While sitting in a good upright position, practice the hundred, noticing the feeling of the belly being scooped up and in by the core muscles.

Practice standing up and sitting down using a good upright chair. Engage the core muscles, lean forward with hands on knees (for balance only) and push up with your legs to standing; then lower yourself down again into the chair. Repeat 5 times, progressing on to 10 when 5 becomes comfortable.

EXERCISE 3

Try to be aware of your core and engage the muscles frequently during different daily activities such as being on public transportation, driving around corners, walking on the flat, up and down hill, up and down stairs, and during sexual intercourse.

EXERCISE 4

Lie on your back on the floor with knees bent up, hips and knees at 90 degrees. Take a deep breath and as you breathe out pull your core in and up and lengthen your left leg away from your body so that when it is straight your left foot should still be at the same height from the floor as your right. While still exhaling draw the left leg back to the starting position. In one breath you extend your leg until straight and return to the starting position. There is no need to hold the leg in the extended position. Repeat with the right leg. Start with 5 repetitions and when comfortable 10 and then 15.

EXERCISE 5

Once you can comfortably do 15 repetitions of exercise 4, the next step is to lower the straightened leg before returning to the starting position. Start by lowering the straightened leg one-third of the height from the floor, then lift again and bend the knee to return to starting position.

Once you are comfortable doing 20 reps you can progress the exercise by lowering two-thirds and then lowering to almost touch the floor.

EXERCISE 6

Plank and side plank. Starting at 2 x 30 seconds and building up in 15-sec increments to 2 x 90 secs.

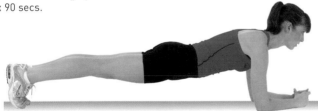

PLANK

Lie in a press-up position, but rest on your forearms, which should be no more than shoulder-width apart, and your toes. Raise your hips until your head, back, and upper legs are in line. Suck in your abs and tense them to hold yourself in position for 15–60 seconds. Slowly lower, rest for 10 seconds and then repeat twice more, keeping your body as still as you can with your abs pulled in, your hips up, and your shoulder blades together.

SIDE PLANK

Lie on your side, supporting your upper body with one elbow and forearm, and your lower body on the side of your foot. Keep your other arm flat against your side (your chest and hips should be at right angles to the floor). Lift your hips so that your spine and legs are in a perfectly straight line and one foot rests on top of the other. Hold yourself perfectly still for 10–30 seconds, then slowly lower your hip to the floor and repeat on the other side.

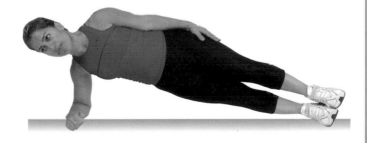

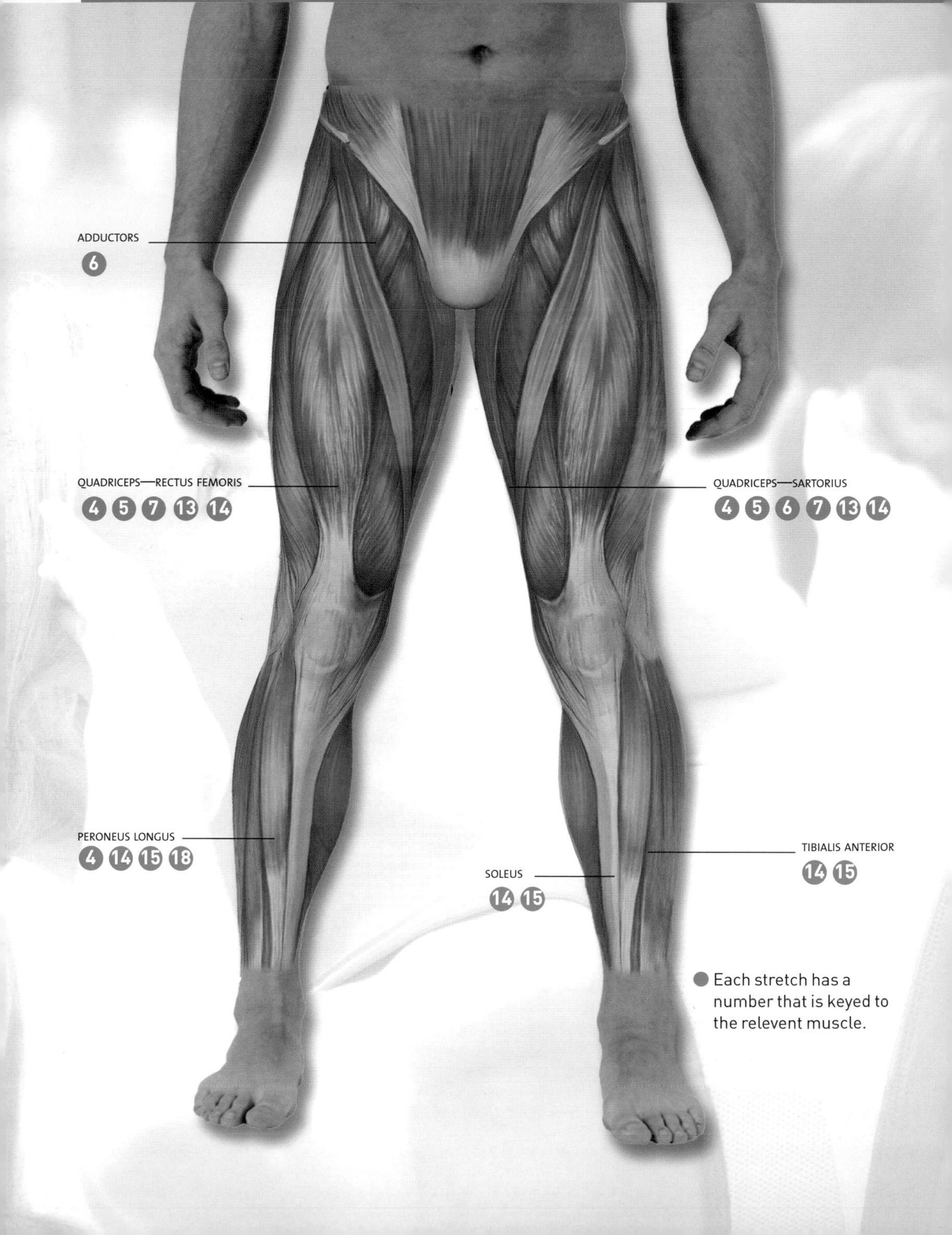

ADDUCTORS
6

QUADRICEPS—RECTUS FEMORIS
4 **5** **7** **13** **14**

QUADRICEPS—SARTORIUS
4 **5** **6** **7** **13** **14**

PERONEUS LONGUS
4 **14** **15** **18**

SOLEUS
14 **15**

TIBIALIS ANTERIOR
14 **15**

● Each stretch has a number that is keyed to the relevent muscle.

GLUTEUS MAXIMUS
8 **9** **11** **15** **16** **18**

HAMSTRINGS
1 **2** **3** **7** **11**

GASTROCNEMIUS
4 **14**

SOLEUS
14 **15** **18**

lower body stretches

There are many activities, such as walking, running, and jumping, that require a degree of fitness from your legs. Achieving fit legs will need a little more effort than just staying active. From the top of the hip to the bottom of the ankle, all the major leg muscles, including the quadriceps, hamstrings, and calves can be flexed and toned with the specifically designed stretches in this section.

TENDON CALCANEUS—ACHILLES

14 **15**

① LYING HAMSTRING STRETCH

Lie flat on the floor. Raise your right leg so that the sole of the foot is resting on the floor and the knee is bent at a 90- degree angle. Slowly raise your left leg, using your hands to help move your thigh back toward your chest and into an upright position. Keep your head relaxed and on the floor throughout the movement. Slowly straighten your left leg in a gentle movement, sliding your hands up toward your calf as the leg extends. Keep your right leg bent to avoid straining your hamstring or lower back. Gently extend your left leg until it is pointing upright. The raise will also put pressure on your lower back—to avoid the vertebrae becoming compressed, do not allow your bottom to lift from the floor. Beginners often overextend—if you feel pain in your extended leg, bend at the

knee to relieve the pressure. To come out of the stretch, reverse the process by gently lowering the leg and allowing the hands to slide down from the calf to the thigh. Now repeat the stretch with the other leg.

If you wish to achieve a greater stretch, use a rolled-up towel around the ankle of the raised leg and pull when the leg is fully extended. Beginners can also use the rolled-up towel to achieve a stretch without compromising the correct posture.

② SEATED HAMSTRING STRETCH

Sit upright with your back straight, your legs extended, and your arms at your sides. Raise your right leg and take the knee out sideways so that it is bent at 90-degrees. Rest the sole of your foot against the inside of your outstretched leg, just below the knee. Bending from the waist, lean forward and reach your hands toward your extended foot. Grasp the foot with both hands, keeping your head facing forward. Pull against the sole of your foot. You will feel a stretch in the hamstrings of your left leg. Pulse the stretch for 10 seconds. Keep the toes pointed forward to ensure the stretch is in the thigh; otherwise, the pull will stay in the shin. Release the stretch, withdraw your hands from your foot, and sit upright. Repeat the stretch on the other leg. Bend forward and perform the stretch on the other side. Remember to keep the toes pointed forward to ensure the stretch is in the thigh, otherwise, the pull will stay in the shin. Pulse the stretch for 10 seconds. You will feel a stretch in the

hamstrings of your right leg. (If you have difficulty reaching the sole of your foot, bend the extended leg slightly to bring the foot closer.) Now raise your head, straighten your back, and extend your left leg in line with the right leg. Place your hands at your sides and relax.

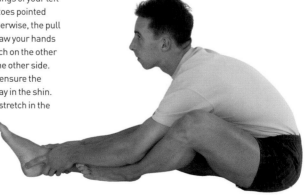

③ STANDING HAMSTRING STRETCH

To perform this exercise, you will need a stool (or similar item) on which to rest your foot and a rolled-up towel to provide support for your ankle. The stool should be roughly waist height. You may also want to stand near a wall for support. Place your weaker leg on the stool with the towel supporting your ankle. Your heel should be resting on the surface of the stool. Your leg can be slightly bent or straight, depending on your flexibility.

Keep your standing leg "soft" and do not lock at the knee. Keep your hips square throughout the exercise to avoid putting pressure on the lower back. Place your hands on either side of your extended knee. Flexing from the waist, slowly bend your body forward, sliding your hands along the leg. Your back should be straight throughout the movement. Keeping your hips square, continue to bend forward until

your hands reach your ankle. If you are flexible enough, extend your arms beyond the ankle to rest your forearms on the towel. Hold the pose.

You will feel a stretch along your hamstring and in your arms as you fully extend. You will also feel a slight stretch in your lower back, which is allowed to arch slightly at the furthest point of the extension. Now slowly reverse the movement, raising up from the waist and sliding your hands back along the leg to return to the start position. Repeat the stretch on the other leg.

For a more extreme stretch, when you are fully extended, shuffle your standing leg away from the stool. To dismount from the stool, shuffle your standing leg forward and bend your outstretched leg until you can easily reach the stool with your hands.

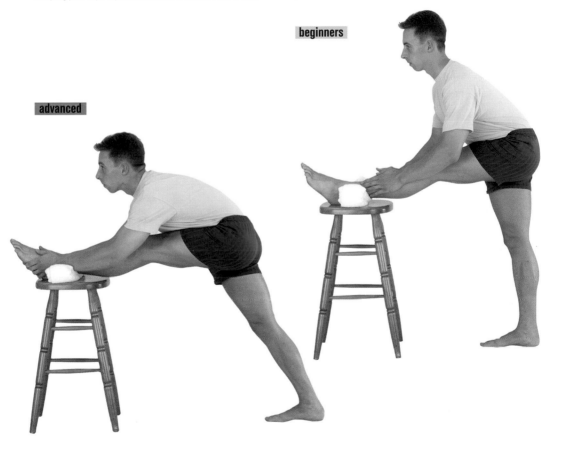

beginners

advanced

④ KNEELING HIP FLEXOR

Begin the exercise with your left leg kneeling on the floor, and your right leg bent at the knee forming a 90-degree angle to the body. Use your hands to push on the right leg to ensure that the head and body are held upright. Keeping your hips facing forward and stomach tucked in, slowly extend your arms forward and allow the fingers to slide along the floor until the palms are pronate. At the same time, extend your left leg away from the body, sliding the toes along the floor. With palms pressed firmly against the floor, gently pulse the left leg to feel a stretch in the upper thigh. Make sure that the hips remain square and facing forward during the stretch, otherwise, the back will arch. Release the stretch and bring your extended arms back into the body. Place your hands back on the right leg. Keep the left leg extended, with the knee resting on the floor. Check that your head and body are upright and the chest is pushed out.

⑤ SEATED ADDUCTOR STRETCH 1

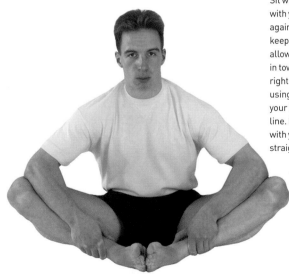

Sit with your legs extended in front and your hands behind you with your palms resting flat on the floor. Press your hands flat against the floor to support the body. Push your chest out, keep your back straight, and keep your elbows soft and do not allow them to lock. Now slowly bend your right leg and bring it in toward the center line of the body. Grip your shin with your right hand to guide the leg inward while maintaining stability using your resting hand. Once the right leg is tucked in, use your left hand to help guide your left leg in toward the center line. Place the soles of your feet together. Now press down with your arms to move your knees apart. Keep your back straight and do not lean forward, as this can strain your lower back. You will feel a stretch along the insides of your thighs. Hold the pose.

⑥ SEATED ADDUCTOR STRETCH 2

This stretch is a progression from adductor stretch 1, once you have placed the soles of your feet together, slowly guide your right leg with your hand facing outward and fully extend at a 45-degree angle. Rest your right hand on your shin. Do the same with your left leg and rest your left hand on your shin. Point your toes outward and stretch your legs as far they will go. If your lower back lacks flexibility, use your arms to press your legs wider apart to achieve a full stretch. Keeping your back upright and shoulders back, breathe deeply and hold the stretch. Release the stretch and bring the legs together again.

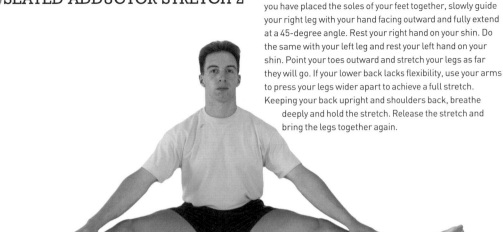

⑦ STANDING QUADRICEPS STRETCH

Stand upright with arms and legs relaxed. Your knees should be quite close together—approximately a hand's-width apart. Slowly flex your left knee and raise your left ankle toward your buttocks while maintaining balance on your standing leg. If you find balancing on one leg difficult, stand near a wall and use your right arm for support. Continue to raise your foot while slowly bringing your left hand back to meet the foot. Hold the foot just below the ankle. Pull the ankle back slightly, but do not bring it back to touch the buttocks, as this can compress the knee joint. Keep your balancing leg slightly bent and soft at the knee—do not lock the knee joint.

To complete the stretch, cup the ankle with your left hand and push your hips slightly forward. Adjust your body weight on to your right leg, push your chest forward, and pull gently on the leg with your left hand. Breathe deeply and hold this position; you will feel a stretch down the front of your upper thigh and hip. Now gently release your ankle and lower the leg to the floor. Repeat the movement with the other leg. Remember that if you cannot easily reach your ankle, you can use a rolled-up towel wrapped around the ankle to help raise the foot.

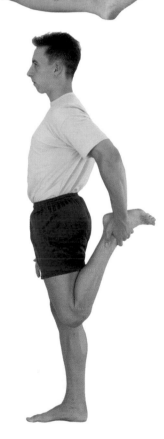

8 SEATED GLUTEAL STRETCH

Sit upright, with both legs extended forward and flat on the floor. Slowly bring your right foot in toward your body, raising your knee into an upright position as you do so. Continue to bring your foot back so that it is level with the knee of the opposite leg. Now use your hands to guide the foot over the opposite knee and rest the sole of the foot on the floor, parallel to and resting against the opposite knee. Wrap both arms around the knee and hug it in toward the chest. Let the knee slot into the angle of the inside of the elbow joint for comfort. The heel of the raised leg should stay on the floor throughout the stretch.

Hold the position and feel a stretch in the gluteal muscles of your right thigh and buttocks. Make sure that the ankle aligns comfortably with the knee to avoid any unpleasant twists as you maintain an upright posture. Release the hug, lift the right foot back over the left leg, and lower the leg to the starting position. Now repeat both stretches using the other leg.

9 GLUTE / PIRIFORMIS STRETCH

Begin this exercise lying flat on your back with your feet spread roughly shoulder-width apart. Place your arms flat on the floor, away from your sides with your palms facing downward. Slowly lift your right knee up to 90 degrees while raising your right hand to rest on the knee. Keep your body straight and back flat against the floor throughout this movement. Now turn your right knee to the left, using your right hand to guide it over your left leg. Turn from the hips, not the lower spine. Keep your left leg extended throughout the movement. Continue to bring the knee down toward the floor, rolling your hips to the left as you do so. It is safe to roll the hips in this exercise because both feet are off the floor, avoiding any unnecessary compression on the back.

Once your right leg is across the left leg, use the left hand to pull the knee down to rest on the floor. Stretch your right arm in the opposite direction to ensure that your shoulders maintain contact with the floor throughout the stretch. Hold the stretch, keeping your knee bent at 90 degrees and your head and chest facing upward. Now release the stretch and bring the leg away from the floor, using your left hand to guide it over your body. Extend your right leg to lie flat and bring your arms down to your sides to return to the starting position. Now perform the stretch on the other side. If you experience any difference in mobility, this may be due to the spinal fluid having moved to the opposite side. Perform the stretch slowly to allow time for the spinal fluid to rebalance itself.

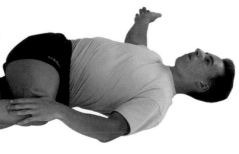

⑩ RAINBOWS   Do not perform this exercise if you have recently suffered a lower back injury.

Lie on your back with your arms extended by your sides and at 90 degrees to the body. Slowly raise your legs, bringing your knees together. Bring your knees up to make a 90-degree angle at the joint. Raise your hands and bring them toward your knees, keeping your back, shoulders, and head flat on the floor. Keeping your knees together, gently push your right knee with your left hand down toward the floor. Pull the knees downward and flat against the floor, using your left hand to apply pressure on the thigh. Stretch your resting arm along the floor and away from the body. This will provide support and ensure that your shoulders remain firmly pressed down. It is important to keep your shoulders pressed

flat on the floor to achieve the correct stretch. Hold the pose for three breaths, pressing the knees to the floor with your left hand, and keeping your head facing upward. You will feel your spine loosen and a stretch along the outside of your thigh. Release the stretch and raise your knees to the upright position with the soles of your feet flat on the floor. Bring your hands back to your sides. Now lower your legs and stretch them out so that they are again flat against the floor. Open your arms outward and rest them against the floor with palms facing upward. Now repeat the stretch on the other side, remembering to keep your shoulders level and against the floor.

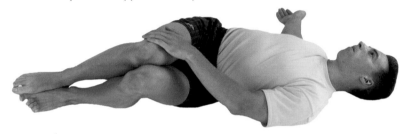

⑪ SINGLE KNEE HUGS

Lie on your back with your legs out straight and your arms rested at your sides. Now slowly raise your left leg bending it at the knee; as you raise and bend your leg reach out with both arms and as the knee gets closer to the chest wrap your arms over it. Pull the knee as close to your chest as possible; to heighten the effect of this stretch simply tighten your arms to hug the knee closer to your chest.

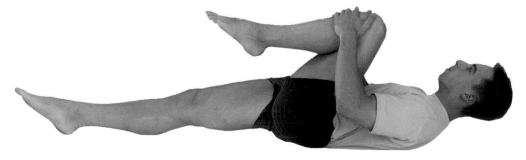

⑫ PELVIC TILTS

Lie on the floor with your knees raised and your feet flat on the floor. There should be a space between the floor and your lower back. Inhale first, then initiate the pelvic tilt movement as you exhale, gently rock your hips toward your face. Your buttocks will not actually leave the floor, but you will feel your lower back press into the floor. An effective pelvic tilt will utilize this leverage begun when the abdomen pulls in during exhale. Just continue the pulling and see how far you can tilt the bottom of your pelvis up. This will result in your lower back gently stretching and reaching in the direction of the floor. Hold this position for a few seconds, then inhale and return to your neutral position. Most of the effort needed to return to the starting position comes from breathing in. Just allow the body to come back to where it began. When performing the pelvic tilt try to pull the pelvis with the abdominals, rather than pushing from the buttocks. Repeat this movement 5 to 10 times.

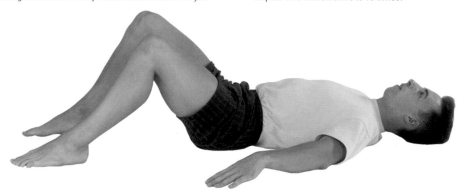

⑬ LYING QUADRICEPS STRETCH

Lying flat on the floor face down, bring your left arm to the front and relax your head on your forearm. To begin the stretch, flex your right leg at the knee and bring the foot toward your buttocks, meeting the ankle with your right hand. Grip your ankle and pull the leg back into the body, so that the heel is roughly 3 inches (8 cm) from the buttocks. Push the hip into the floor to lift the knee from the ground to increase the stretch. You will feel a stretch in your quadriceps and along the outside of your right hip. Hold the position for a few breaths. Now release the leg. Extend your leg back toward the floor so that it is lying flat. Repeat the stretch on the other side.

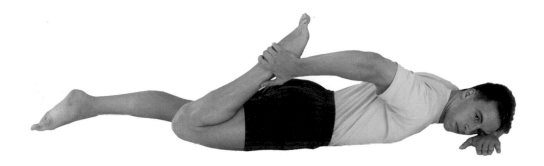

⑭ SQUATS

Stand with feet about hip- or shoulder-width apart. Contract the abs and keep them tight as you bend the knees and slowly squat down. Keeping the knees behind the toes, continue the squat until your thighs are parallel to the floor, your knees at 90 degrees. Hold this position for a few seconds, then still contracting the glutes and hamstrings lift and begin extending the legs. Fully extend the legs until you're back to standing position. Always keep the knees in line with the toes.

Once you're comfortable doing squats, it's time to progress and add some challenge to them. There are several options, such as holding a dumbell in each hand outside your thighs. This is a great way to add intensity without putting any extra load onto the spine.

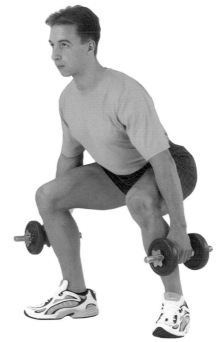

⑮ ONE-LEGGED SQUAT

Stand with your back to a bench or a chair. Shift your balance so that you're standing on one leg and carefully place the foot of your other leg on the bench or chair. Keeping your hips level and your hands on your hips, your back straight, slowly bend your knee until your hamstring is parallel to the floor. Tip your hips forward and push up with your thigh to slowly straighten your leg. The slower and more controlled you do this squat the more effective it is. Remember when doing squats that the knee of the weight-bearing leg should never come forward of your toes.

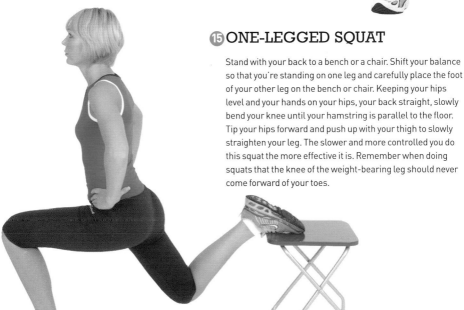

⑯ PRONE PIGEON

From a lunge stretch position with right leg forward and the left knee and hands on the floor, bring the right foot across outside of the left hand and lower the knee in front of the body allowing the foot to roll onto its side. As you go forward allow your pelvis to bring your left thigh down to the mat. If you are comfortable like this with your hands still supporting the position, you can bring your trunk forward so that you are lying on your bent knee. Repeat on the other side.

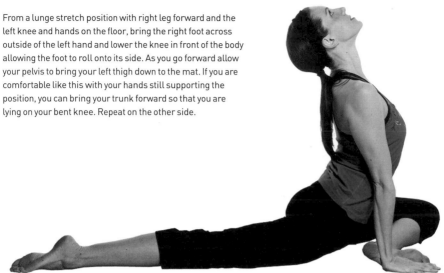

⑰ FEET DOWN KNEE ROTATION

Lie on your back with knees bent up, feet on floor, and arms outstretched to the side. While turning your head to the left let your knees fall out to the right until the right thigh touches the floor. Its okay for the pelvis to roll over. Then bring your knees back up through the midline and allow them to fall out to the left while turning the head to the right. Repeat using your hip abdomen and back muscles to keep the movement smooth.

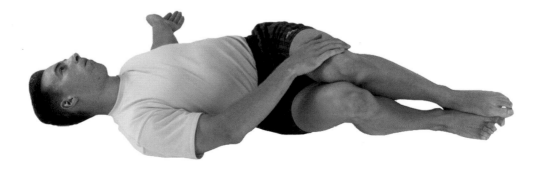

18 DEEP SQUAT STRETCH

Stand with feet about hip- or shoulder-width apart.
Contract the abs and keep them tight as you bend the knees
and slowly squat down. Keeping the knees behind the toes
continue the squat until your thighs are parallel to the floor,
your knees at 90 degrees. At the same time as you are
lowering into the squat reach up with both arms and stretch
them above your head. Hold this position for a few seconds,
then still contracting the glutes and hamstrings lift and
begin extending the legs. Fully extend the legs until you're
back to standing position. Always keep the knees in line
with the toes.

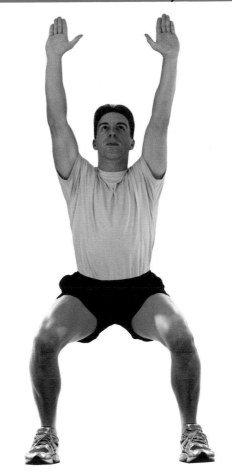

19 PRONE TRUNK RAISE

Lie on your front with arms by your sides. Use your back
muscles to lift your upper body off the floor in a controlled
movement. Lift up as far as is comfortable and lower to the
floor again in good control. Repeat.

20 TRUNK RAISE HANDS AT HEAD

As with the prone trunk raise, lie on your front, but this time
place your hands touching each side of your head. Use your
back muscles to lift your upper body off the floor in a
controlled movement. Lift up as far as is comfortable and
lower to the floor again in good control. Repeat.

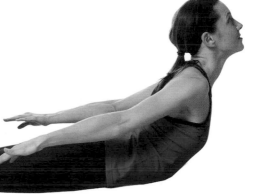

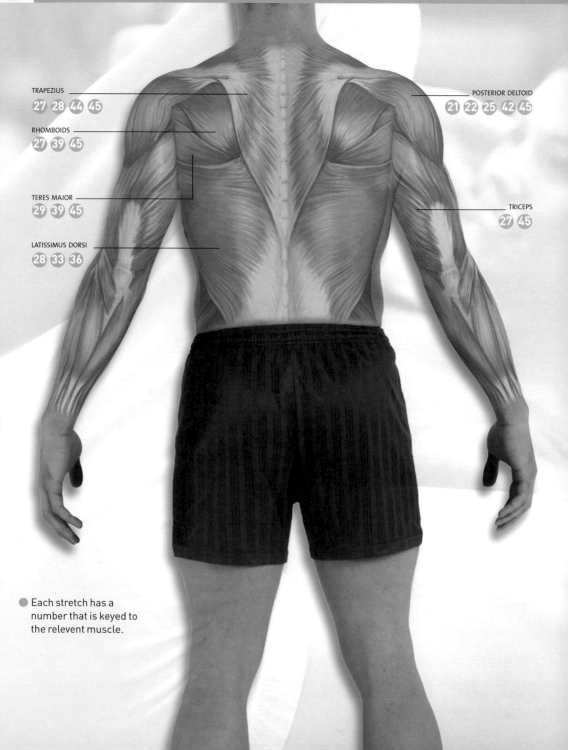

TRAPEZIUS
27 28 44 45

RHOMBOIDS
27 39 45

TERES MAJOR
29 39 45

LATISSIMUS DORSI
28 33 36

POSTERIOR DELTOID
21 22 25 42 45

TRICEPS
27 45

Each stretch has a number that is keyed to the relevent muscle.

upper body stretches

This section concentrates on stretches to tone and flex the muscles of the upper body, arms, and the abdomen.

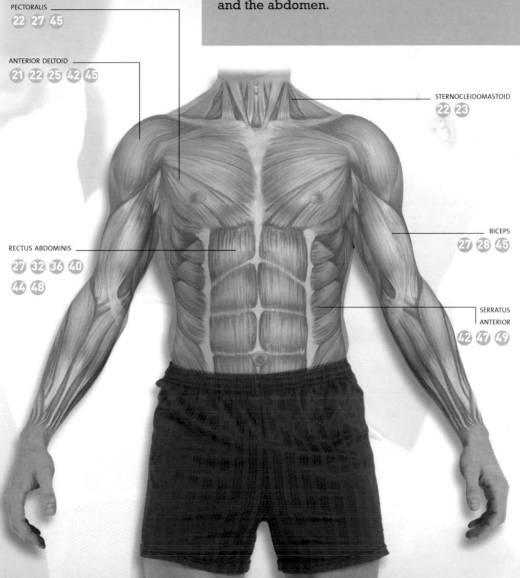

PECTORALIS
22 **27** **45**

ANTERIOR DELTOID
21 **22** **25** **42** **45**

STERNOCLEIDOMASTOID
22 **23**

BICEPS
27 **28** **45**

RECTUS ABDOMINIS
27 **32** **36** **40**
44 **48**

SERRATUS
ANTERIOR
42 **47** **49**

㉑ ARM RAISES ABOVE HEAD

Stand with your feet roughly shoulder-width apart and your arms hanging loosely at your sides. Keep your legs soft at the knees. Inhale and slowly raise your arms, keeping them straight at the elbow. Move the arms in an upward movement that expands outward from the center. You should be fully inhaled as your hands reach head height. With your palms facing outward, extend your hands toward the sky, facing your head forward as you do. Exhale as your hands reach skyward, and hold this position for a few seconds. Now reverse the downward movement, exhale, and slowly lower your arms. Bring your arms back to your sides and relax your body.

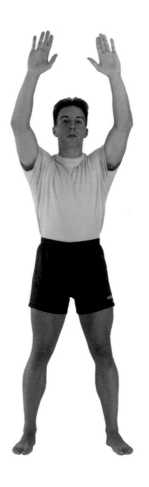

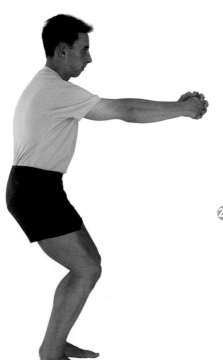

㉒ ARM RAISES IN FRONT

Stand with your feet roughly shoulder-width apart and your arms hanging loosely at your sides. Keep your legs soft at the knees. Inhale and slowly raise your arms, crossing them as they pass in front of your chest. Move the arms in an upward movement that expands outward from the center. You should be fully inhaled as your hands reach head height. With your palms facing outward, extend your hands toward the sky, facing your head forward as you do. Exhale as your hands reach skyward, and hold this position for a few seconds. Now reverse the downward movement, exhale, and slowly lower your arms. Bring your arms back to your sides and relax your body.

㉓ STANDING NECK STRETCH

Stand upright with your feet shoulder-width apart and your arms relaxed at your sides, palms facing behind you. Raise your left hand up toward your head and move your right arm behind your back so that the elbow is at 90 degrees and the forearm is resting in the small of your back. Bring your raised hand over your head to grasp the right side of your crown. Relax your neck muscles and gently pull down with the hand, keeping your body upright. Keep the movement isolated to the neck. Continue the stretch by gently pulling downward and forward with your right arm. For safety, do not pull or push the head suddenly or move it into a position that is uncomfortable. Release the head, switch over hands, and repeat the process on the other side, remembering to keep your neck relaxed throughout. Now release the stretch and bring both arms to rest at your sides.

㉔ STANDING NECK ROTATION

Stand upright with your feet positioned shoulder-width apart and your arms relaxed at your sides. Turn your head to the left until you feel the stretch in your neck, hold for a few seconds, then slowly release back to the center. Repeat on the other side.

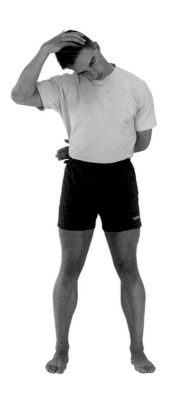

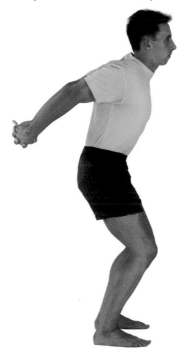

㉕ ARM RAISES BEHIND

Stand with your feet spaced no more than shoulder-width apart. Keep the knees soft and make sure that they do not lock during the stretch. Now slowly take your arms behind the body and clasp the hands together by interlocking your fingers. Bend the knees gently, and lean the upper body forward. Remember to keep the back straight as the body lowers; otherwise, the stretch in the chest will be lost. Push your buttocks away from the midline. Raise the arms to feel a stretch across the chest; you will feel a stretch in the front of the shoulders too as the arms get higher. At full stretch, exhale and then bend forward to pulse the movement. Release the stretch and bring the arms back toward the body. Unclasp the hands and let them fall to the sides. Gently straighten the body into the upright position, making sure that the hips are square, the chest is pushed out, and the head is held up.

26 SPHINX

Start by lying on your front with your legs straight back and pressing the top of your feet into the floor. The entire length of your legs needs to be firmly grounded into the floor. To really feel this, lengthen each leg back through your toes and turn your thighs a little more inward—you should now feel the entire front of your legs in contact with the floor. Now, place your elbows directly under your shoulders with your forearms straight in front of your body. With the palms facing down spread your fingers wide and feel the weight of your upper-body spread through your forearms and out through each finger. Now start to stretch the spine. On an in-breath, begin to push weight into your hands while sliding your shoulder blades down your back; as you raise push out your chest between your arms. As your chest grows upward, your spine will begin to lengthen, and your hips are grounded, so bringing your chest forward will lengthen your spine. Stay for a few breaths. If you feel pain in your lower back, try relaxing the bend. On the exhalation, lower yourself to the starting position.

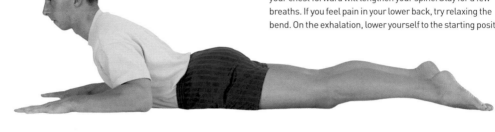

27 PUSH-UPS

Kneel on the floor with your hands about two shoulder-widths apart. Extend your legs behind you, keeping your back and legs straight and your head in line with your body, and rest your toes the floor. Inhale as you slowly lower yourself by bending your arms, without letting your hips drop, until your chest brushes the floor. Exhale as you push back up by straightening your arms. Keep your hips and legs in line with your spine.

28 PUSH-UPS WITH CLAPPING

Kneel on the floor with your hands about two shoulder-widths apart. Extend your legs behind you, keeping your back and legs straight and your head in line with your body, and rest your toes the floor. Inhale as you slowly lower yourself by bending your arms, without letting your hips drop, until your chest brushes the floor. Exhale as you push hard and fast so as to explode up from the floor, as your hands leave the floor clap them together before landing back with both hands.

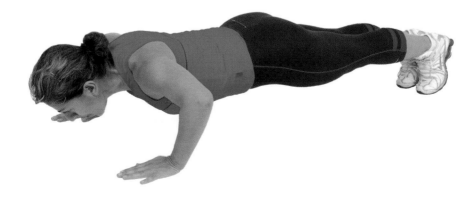

29 UNDER / OVER HAND CLASP

Stand with your feet shoulder-width apart, bring your right hand over your head and down your back between your shoulder blades. Bring your left hand up behind your back and clasp the hands together to stretch the shoulders and upper arms. If you can't reach, hold a rolled-up towel in your right hand and grasp it with the left. Swap hands and repeat. You may find that your shoulders are not evenly mobile; don't worry, just work a little more on the stiffer side.

30 PRONE SUPERMAN below

Lie on your front on the floor, with your arms outstretched above your head and your legs extended, with your feet slightly apart and your hands shoulder-width apart. Breathe in as you simultaneously raise your right arm and left leg off the floor by contracting the muscles of your lower back and bottom. Hold for 5–15 seconds, then slowly lower and repeat with the left arm and right leg. Take care not to twist your spine or overstress your back.

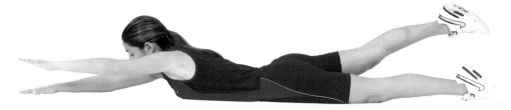

31 CRUCIFIX STRETCH

Stand with arms lifted up out to the side at shoulder level, stretching right out to the fingertips. Turn the right hand palm up and the left turned down, head turned to the right. Take a deep breath and as you breathe out slowly turn your palms so that the left is up and the right is down. At the same time slowly turn your head to the left so that you always look at the upturned palm. Repeat.

32 ONE-LEGGED BRIDGE below

Lie on your back with your arms by your sides. Bend one knee and bring your foot in so that your calf almost touches the back of your thigh. Leave the other leg extended flat along the floor. Keeping your arms, head, and shoulders on the floor and the extended leg straight, push your hips into the air until your chest, stomach, hips, and knees are in line. Hold this raised position for 15–45 seconds, then lower yourself to the starting position and repeat twice more for each side.

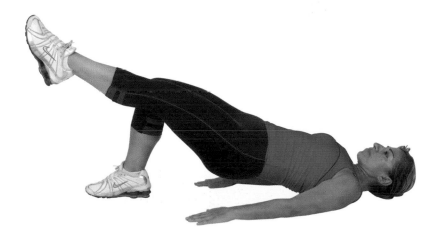

33 COBRA

Begin the exercise kneeling on the floor with your body upright and your arms relaxed at your sides. Your knees should be close together but not touching, with your feet pointing away from your body. Now lean forward, bending from the waist, and bring your arms down to rest the palms flat on the floor. Keep your back straight throughout the forward bend. Walk your hands forward and continue to extend your body. Lower your hips to the ground while keeping your upper body raised with the palms of your hands. Let the lower body sink to create an inverse arch in the back. Keep your head up and face forward. Hold the pose briefly, pulsing the stretch by pressing down with the palms. Release the pose and lift yourself off the floor and back on to your hands and knees, with your back straight and hips aligned.

34 COBRA INTO UPWARD DOG

From the cobra pose continue pushing upward with your arms, while arching your back. Your arms should be absolutely straight and the only parts of your body touching the floor should be your hands and the tops of your feet.

35 CHALK CIRCLES

Lie on your left side with your right knee bent up in front of you and your shoulder forward and left hand on your right knee. Your head, body, and left leg should be in a straight line. Stretch your right hand forward as far as you can to touch the floor and then bring your hand down toward your legs keeping it stretched out as far as possible. Imagine trying to draw as big a circle as possible on the floor keeping the hand as low as possible all the way round. If you find it uncomfortable on the shoulder, lift your arm to go around the painful part of the arc, don't try to go through the pain. Draw three clockwise circles and three counterclockwise and then turn over and repeat on the other side.

36 CAT INTO COW

Lie flat with your legs outstretched and your forearms and the palms of your hands flat against the floor with your elbows out at the sides. Your head should be rested on the floor between your hands. Now slowly raise your head and push against the floor with your hands to lift your chest from the floor. Flexing at the knees, lift your hips from the floor to bring yourself up onto all fours with your arms locked at the elbows. Face down toward the floor. All your weight should now be on your hands and knees. Walk your hands backward a few inches to arch your back upward in the Cat pose. Hold the pose and pulse the stretch by bending your head inward. Now release the stretch and lift your head up while simultaneously pushing your buttocks outward. Push your chest down to gain an inverted arch in the back. Hold the pose for a few seconds. You will feel a stretch in your lower back.

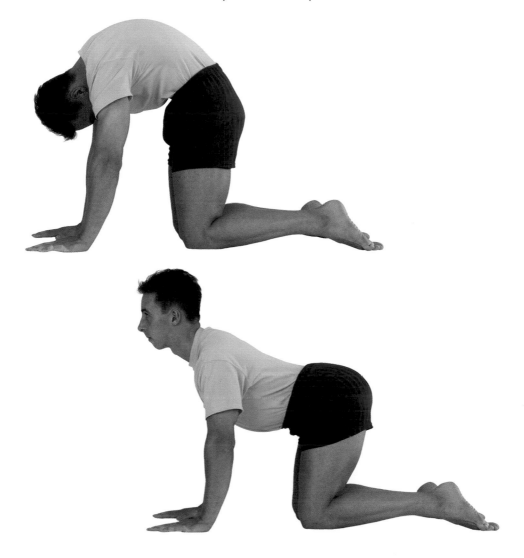

③⑦ SUPERMAN

Start by getting down on your hands and knees. You can make this superman exercise more comfortable by placing a folded towel underneath your knees. Next, tighten your abdominal muscles and focus and control your breathing. Push your hands into the floor and push your back up toward the ceiling, so you can feel the squeeze in the muscles of your upper back. While maintaining this squeeze in your upper back, raise your left arm and right leg to form the superman position. Your left arm through to your right leg should be parallel to the ground. You are now in the kneeling superman position. If you find it difficult to maintain your balance, then for the first couple of days only raise your arm and leave your knees on the ground. Hold this superman position for 5 breaths. Return to the start position. Repeat the superman exercise, but this time raise the right arm and left leg. Complete the full superman exercise by repeating 5 times, remembering to alternate your arms and legs. Once you are comfortable doing the superman exercise you can make it more difficult by increasing the number of repetitions and also gradually increase the 5 breath hold to 15 breath holds.

③⑧ CAMEL

Start this exercise as you finished the Cat sequence, kneeling on all fours with your hands roughly in line with your shoulders and your back straight and level with the floor. Flexing at the knees, gradually lower your hips toward your heels, stretching your back, shoulders, and arms as you do so.

Extend your arms and point your fingers away from the body. Hold the stretch. Slide your hands backward toward your knees and slowly raise your torso into an upright seated position. Bring your hands on fingertips past your legs and sit upright. Push your chest forward. Continue to slide your hands backward until they are level with your feet and your buttocks are resting on your heels. Move your hands back behind your feet and rest your palms flat on the floor. Arch your chest upward and take your body weight on your arms.

Slowly roll the head back so that your chin points upward at 90 degrees to the floor. Gently flex your hips and pelvis forward to gain a full stretch. Hold the pose. You will feel a stretch in the abdomen and hips. Release the stretch. Supporting yourself on your hands, lower your hips and bring your chest forward to straighten your body. Return to an upright, seated posture with your buttocks resting on your heels. Now lift your body from the knees, leaning forward to come out of the seated position. Finish kneeling upright, with your arms relaxed, your back straight, and your head facing forward.

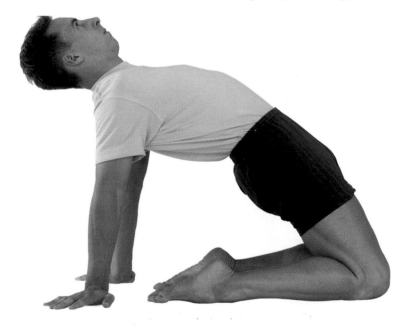

39 DOWNWARD DOG

Come onto the floor on your hands and knees. Set your knees directly below your hips and your hands slightly forward of your shoulders. Spread your palms, index fingers parallel or slightly turned out, and turn your toes under. Exhale and lift your knees away from the floor. At first keep the knees slightly bent and the heels lifted away from the floor. Lengthen your tailbone away from the back of your pelvis and press it lightly toward the pubis. Against this resistance, lift the sitting bones toward the ceiling, and from your inner ankles draw the inner legs up into the groins. Then with an exhalation, push your top thighs back and stretch your heels onto or down toward the floor. Straighten your knees but be sure not to lock them. Firm the outer thighs and roll the upper thighs inward slightly. Narrow the front of the pelvis. Firm the outer arms and press the bases of the index fingers actively into the floor. From these two points lift along your inner arms from the wrists to the tops of the shoulders. Firm your shoulder blades against your back, then widen them and draw them toward the tailbone. Keep the head between the upper arms; don't let it hang. Stay in this pose anywhere from 1 to 3 minutes. Then bend your knees to the floor with an exhalation and rest.

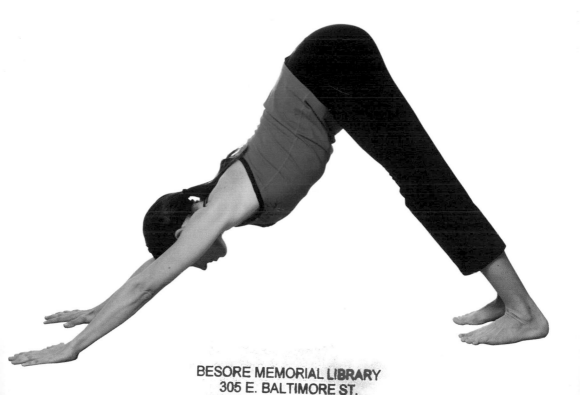

④⓪ WALKING LUNGES

Standing tall with your shoulders back and down and abdominals engaged, place your feet together. Your arms can be flat at your side, holding your hips or behind your head. Breathing normally, step forward with your right foot, bending both knees so that your front knee is aligned over your ankle and the back knee comes close to the floor. Your back heel is lifted off the floor. Before your back knee touches the floor, push up with your back left leg, forcing the weight of your body through your right heel, simultaneously bringing your left foot together with your right foot. Without pausing, alternate legs, lunge forward with your left foot, bending both knees so that your front knee is aligned with your ankle and the back knee comes close to the floor. Your back heel is lifted off the floor. Before your back knee touches the floor, push up with your back right leg, forcing the weight of your body through your left heel, simultaneously bringing your right foot together with your left foot. Continue to perform the steps above, alternating legs for 20 steps and increasing the steps as you get stronger.

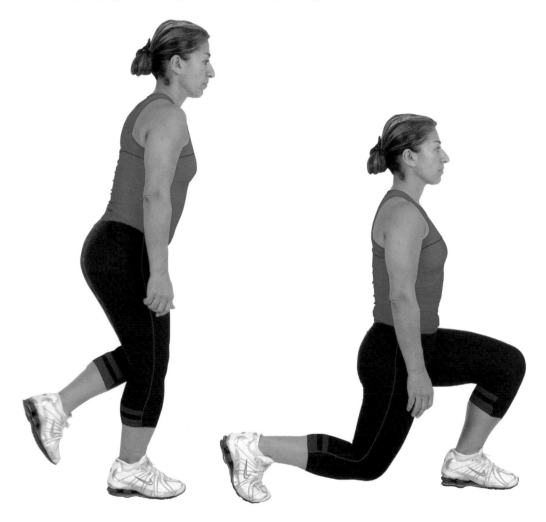

41 STANDING FORWARD BEND

Stand with your legs together and your weight centered on the balls of your feet. Inhale, and stretch both of your arms straight up overhead, alongside your ears. Keeping your legs straight, exhale and bend forward at the waist, reaching down and grabbing hold of the back of your legs wherever it feels the most comfortable. As you gain flexibility in your legs, try different holds to get different stretches—looping your fingers around your big toes, sliding your fingers and palms under the front of your feet, or catching hold of your elbows behind your legs. Keep your head and neck relaxed, allowing gravity to do its work. Hold the pose, breathing smoothly and evenly for several breaths. As you get more comfortable with this pose, you'll be able to stay in it for minutes at a time. Release the pose by bringing your hands to your hips, lifting the straight torso to waist level so it's parallel to the floor, and then raising it up straight on an inhale.

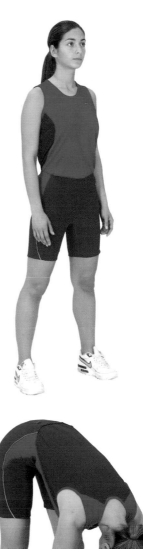

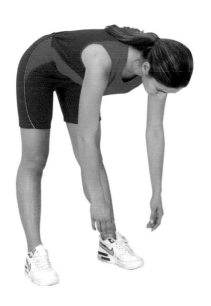

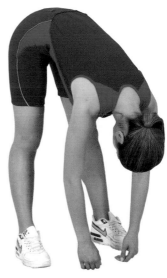

42 LUNGE HANDS UP

From a standing position, feet shoulder-width apart, take a large step forward with your right leg. Start by placing your hands on your hips, slowly lower your left knee toward the floor, bending your right leg at the knee; keep your back nice and straight and make sure that your right knee does not go over your toe. Now exhale as you push up with your right leg, and exhale as you lower yourself down again. Once you feel balanced raise both arms straight over your head and lunge 10 to 15 times, then repeat the lunge on the left side.

43 LUNGE HANDS FORWARD

As with the previous lunge but with your arms raised straight out in front of you, palms of the hands facing down. This may be a little easier to practice if you are not confidently balanced with your arms above your head.

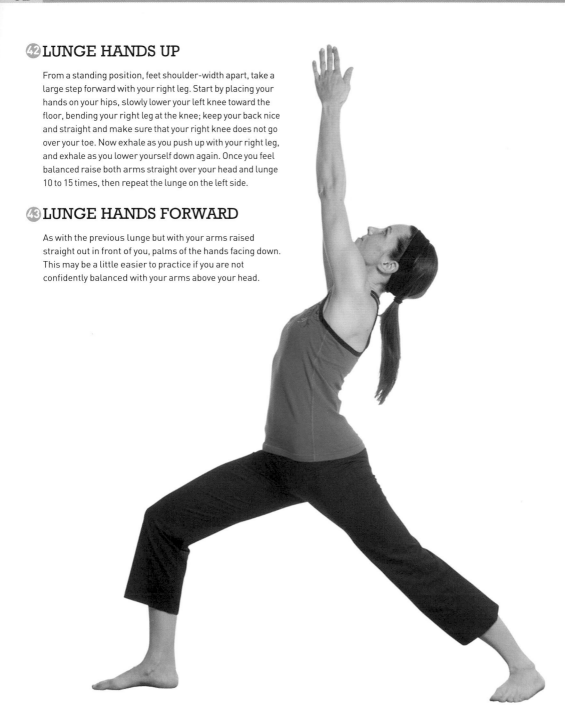

44 STRAIGHT LEG RAISE

Lying on your back with your arms by your sides and your legs outstretched, pull your stomach muscles in. Breathe out as you lift your legs off the floor until your toes are directly over your hips. Try to roll your lower back off the floor using your abs. Very slowly, lower both legs until your feet hover just above the floor, then repeat.

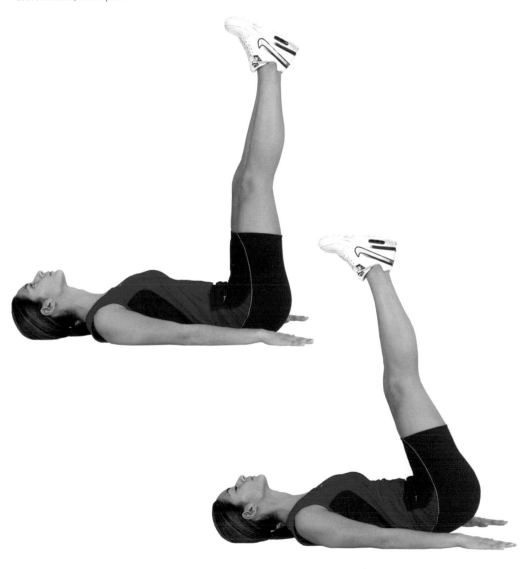

④⑤ RAISED PUSH-UPS

Kneel on the floor with a chair behind you and your hands
about two shoulder-widths apart. Extend your legs behind
you, keeping your back and legs straight and your head in line
with your body. Rest your toes on the step. Inhale as you
slowly lower yourself by bending your arms, without letting
your hips drop, until your chest brushes the floor. Exhale as
you push back up by straightening your arms. Keep your hips
and legs in line with your spine.

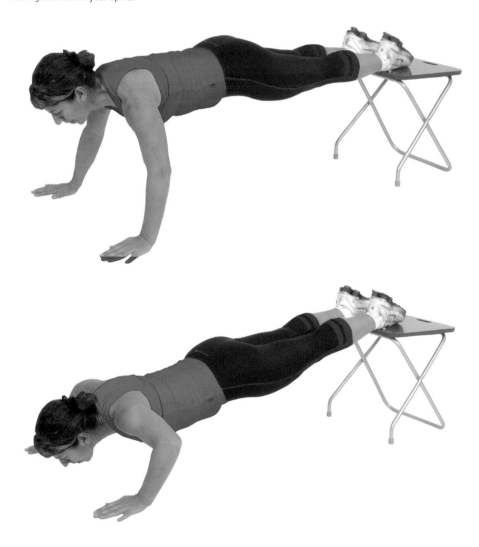

46 STANDING WARRIOR 1

Start the sequence from the Downward Dog asana (see p 49), with your feet and hands pressed firmly on the ground and your hips raised in the air so that your body forms an inverted "V" shape. Slowly, raise your right leg, lifting from the toes of your left foot. Bring your right leg underneath and into your body so that your knee is beneath your chest. Maintain balance with your fingers pressed into the floor and arms locked at the elbows. Now slowly straighten your back and raise your head. Simultaneously, lower your hips toward the floor and stretch your left leg to fully extend. Rest your left knee and the fingertips of both hands on the floor.Slowly raise and outstretch your arms. Bring your hands together, joining at the palms. Tilt your head backward and gradually arch your back. Continue to reach up toward the sky until your face and arms are pointed vertically. Hold the pose for three breaths, breathing deeply. You will feel a stretch in your shoulders and back, and in your groin and thighs. Slowly reverse the process to come out of the stretch.

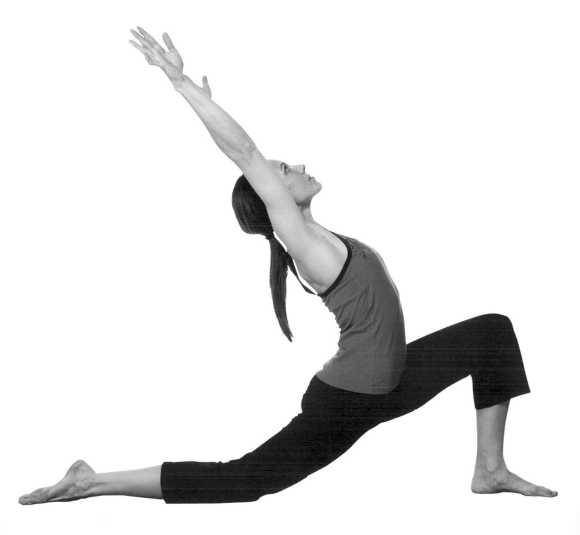

47 STANDING WARRIOR 2

An additional stretch to the warrior position, lower your body toward your left knee, placing your left hand on the floor beside your left foot. Now slowly raise your right arm up and over your head, and you will feel a stretch down your right-hand side. Turn your head to look up to your raised arm and hold the stretch for a few seconds; slowly reverse the movement to come out of the stretch. Repeat on the other side.

48 STANDING WARRIOR 3

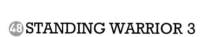

This stretch is all about balance. Starting in Warrior I position, bring your hands to your hips. Now move your weight to your right foot and raise your left foot from the floor. Bring your torso forward, aligning it so that it is parallel with the floor. Relax your neck. Bring your back, raised leg in line with the rest of your body. Make sure your hips are pointed to the floor. Flex your raised foot. Bring your arms to your side. Hold for 30 seconds to a minute. Release back to the lunge as you exhale. Repeat on the other side. If you have trouble balancing, you can use a chair to support your arms.

49 STANDING TRIANGLES

Spread your feet apart by about 40 inches (1 meter), with toes pointing forward. Extend your arms out from your sides so that they are parallel with the floor and level with your shoulders. Keep your palms facing toward the floor. Slowly turn your right foot to an angle of 90 degrees so that it is pointing in the same direction as your extended right arm. Turn your other foot 30 degrees to the right. Keep your feet flat on the floor. Square the hips so that they are facing forward, together with your chest and head.

Hinging from the lower body, slowly reach down to your right. Turning your head to face to the right, bring your extended right hand down to rest on your shin just below the knee. The movement should cause your left arm to become vertical and point skyward. This pose should create a straight line from your foot to the end of your extended left hand. Look up toward your right hand. Hold the pose for eight breaths. You will feel a stretch in your spine, along the left side of your torso and across the shoulders.

⑤⓪ STANDING SPINE ROTATION

Stand upright with your feet facing forward and spaced roughly shoulder-width apart. Keep your knees soft and do not lock the joints. Slowly bring your hands out to the front of your chest. Bend your elbows and extend them so that they are parallel to the floor. Place one hand on top of the other so that they are crossed at the wrists. Bend slightly at the knees and maintain a straight and upright back. Holding your arms steady, rotate the upper body from the waist to your left side. Turn your head in rotation with your body. Keep your hips facing forward throughout the rotation to ensure that all the movement is in the muscles of the upper body. Your hips, knees, and feet

should form a sturdy base for the rotation. Continue the stretch as far as possible without turning your hips. Turn your head as far as you can to attain a stretch in the neck. Keep your knees soft and your feet facing forward. Hold the pose briefly. Now release the stretch and rotate the body to the opposite side. Make the movement slowly to avoid damaging your spine or back muscles. Repeat the stretch, remembering to keep your feet facing forward and your hips square throughout. Now return your body to the starting position, bring your feet together, and lower your arms back to the sides of your body. You can repeat this exercise until tired.

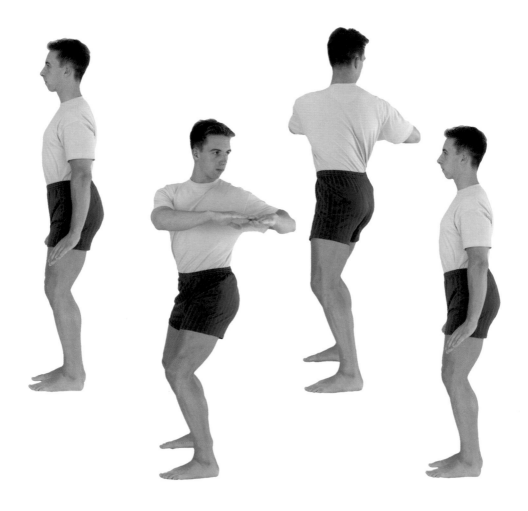

⑤⑪ STANDING FULL-LEG STRETCH

For safety, when doing this stretch do not force the leg any higher than feels comfortable. Begin the exercise standing upright, with your feet spaced shoulder-width apart and facing forward. Slowly lift your right leg, shifting your weight to your left side. Lift your leg with the sole of your foot coming inward toward your thigh. Reach down to grasp your ankle with your right hand. Keep the other arm extended to remain steady and maintain balance. Hold the sole of your foot so that it is resting against the inside of the opposite thigh, just above the knee. Now slowly extend the leg away from the body, using your hand to aid a smooth extension. Take the leg out to its full extent and grip the sole of the foot to bring the leg up to about head height. Concentrate on straightening the leg before reaching up for a greater angle.

You will feel a stretch along the inside of your extended thigh. Exhale and hold the pose. At full stretch push your hips and chest forward. To maintain balance, lean your body slightly to the left with your left arm extended. Do not let the standing leg lock, but remain flexible. If you are holding your leg at waist height, the guiding hand should be around the ankle; if you have achieved a higher raise, hold the outside of the raised foot. Gently lower your leg, using your hand to aid a smooth movement. Use your other arm to maintain good balance and keep your standing leg soft at the knee for flexibility. Return to the standing position, with your arms relaxed at your sides. Now repeat the stretch on the other leg, remembering not to cause injury by forcing an excessive extension.

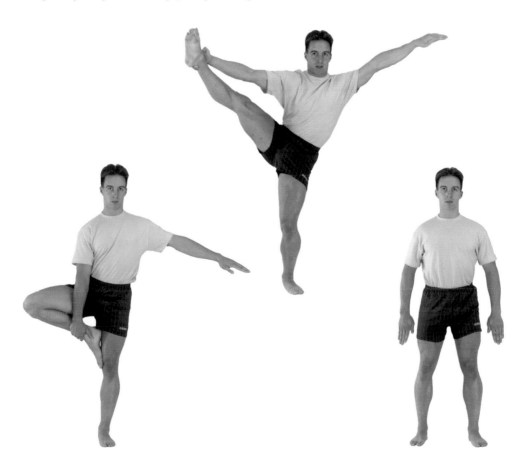

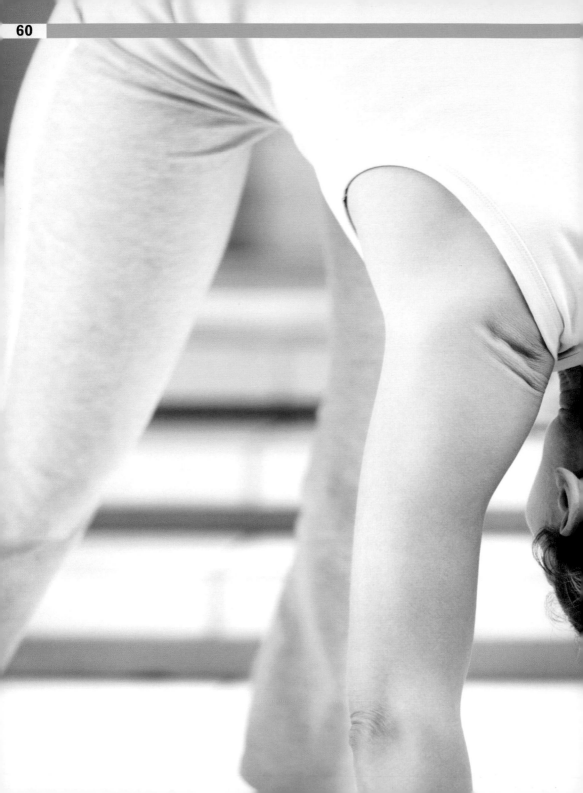

stretching schedules

One of the key factors to getting the most out of exercising and making progress is to follow a schedule. This does not mean subjecting yourself to strict regimes or subscribing to detailed instructions and rules. It simply means giving yourself a working framework and goals to aim for that are achievable. Following a basic plan will help you to keep motivated and achieve your goals.

This chapter provides day-by-day guides at six levels of fitness and ability, designed to help you achieve a wide range of stretching and fitness goals safely and effectively.

how the stretching levels work

The training schedules in this section are divided into six levels of difficulty. The levels can be used alone or followed consecutively, and each includes higher cardiovascular intensity and deeper stretches than the last. The first training level is purely for beginners. Its purpose is to build you up to walking, cycling, or swimming for 20 minutes nonstop. All the other levels feature a fitness-running schedule, and one or more racing schedules. The levels are arranged like this:

1 STARTER LEVEL

PAGES 64–67
for absolute beginners

The schedule aims to:

start building strength and increase your flexibility

enable you to run, cycle, or swim for 20 minutes

It is a flexible schedule that lasts for 8 weeks.

Perform each stretch once unless indicated.

2 STARTER LEVEL

PAGES 68–71
for those returning to exercise or relatively new to exercise

for increasing your strength and flexibility

enable you to run, cycle, or swim for 30 minutes

Perform each stretch once unless indicated.

3 INTERMEDIATE LEVEL

PAGES 72–75
for those who are active but not in regular exercise

for focusing activity and progression

enable you to run, cycle, or swim for 30–40 minutes

Perform each stretch once unless indicated.

BE CAREFUL

Remember that all of the following schedules are guidelines only, and each schedule is intended for people of the appropriate fitness level. Do not push yourself excessively, and listen to your body—if you feel any serious pain or discomfort, especially if you have not exercised regularly over the last five years, consult a doctor or sports injury specialist immediately.

4 INTERMEDIATE LEVEL	**5** UPPER LEVEL	**6** UPPER LEVEL
PAGES 76–79	PAGES 80–85	PAGES 86–93
for those exercising 2–3 times per week	**for those exercising 3–4 times per week**	**for those exercising 5–7 times per week**
for increasing strength, flexibility, and general fitness, and introducing speedwork (intervals) to the schedules	for increasing strength and flexibility, and to reduce training injuries	for maximizing the benefits of training routines and increasing strength and flexibility
enable you to run, cycle, or swim for 40 minutes plus	enable you to run, cycle, or swim for 50 minutes plus	enable you to run, cycle, or swim for 75 minutes
Perform each stretch once unless indicated.	Perform each stretch once unless indicated.	Perform each stretch once unless indicated.

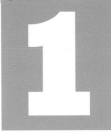

starter level 1

This schedule is aimed at absolute beginners, people who have had no regular exercise, people returning from injury or a long lay off from exercise. The aim is to increase movement with confidence, reducing aches and pains. Let's get moving!

WEEK	MONDAY	TUESDAY	WEDNESDAY	
1	daily stretch (p14) 20-minute walk at a comfortable pace	daily stretch (p14) 20-minute walk at a comfortable pace	daily stretch (p14) 20-minute walk at a comfortable pace	
2	daily stretch (p14), 20-minute walk, supine hamstring stretch, rainbows 5x, glute/piriformis stretch, forward/backward arm arc 5x, Cat into Cow 5x	daily stretch (p14) 20-minute walk at a comfortable pace	daily stretch (p14), 20-minute cardio, supine hamstring stretch, rainbows 5x, glute/piriformis stretch, forward/backward arm arc 5x, Cat into Cow 5x	
3	daily stretch (p14) supine hamstring stretch, rainbows 5x, glute/piriformis stretch, forward/backward arm arc 5x, Cat into Cow 5x, seated hamstring stretch, glute stretch, chest stretch arms in front, arms behind, repeat with straight arms above head	daily stretch (p14) 20-minute walk at a comfortable pace	daily stretch (p14) supine hamstring stretch, rainbows 5x, glute/piriformis stretch, forward/backward arm arc 5x, Cat into Cow 5x, seated hamstring stretch, glute stretch, chest stretch arms in front, arms behind, repeat with straight arms above head	
4	daily stretch (p14) supine hamstring stretch, rainbows 5x, glute/piriformis stretch, forward/backward arm arc 5x, Cat into Cow 5x, seated hamstring stretch, glute stretch, chest stretch arms in front, arms behind, repeat with straight arms above head	daily stretch (p14) and 20-minute walk, 20–30 minutes of running, cycling, swimming, or rowing at a steady pace	daily stretch (p14) supine hamstring stretch, rainbows 5x, glute/piriformis stretch, forward/backward arm arc 5x, Cat into Cow 5x, seated hamstring stretch, glute stretch, chest stretch arms in front, arms behind, repeat with straight arms above head	

WEEK 4—PICK UP THE CARDIO

This week we will introduce some structured cardiovascular exercise: walking, cycling, or swimming, whatever you enjoy and can most easily fit into your week. 20-minutes 2–3 times per week of activity that doesn't make you breathless, but begins to make you sweat. If you can't manage 20 minutes in one session, then break it down into smaller sessions.

REMEMBER—GENTLY DOES IT!

If you are not used to regular exercising and can't do 20 minutes walking, start with what you feel comfortable with, 3 minutes perhaps. As you progress add 1, 2, or 3 minutes each day until you have achieved the 20 minutes. Likewise with the stretches; just do the daily stretches until you are comfortable adding more to your program.

THURSDAY	FRIDAY	SATURDAY	SUNDAY
daily stretch (p14) 20-minute walk at a comfortable pace	daily stretch (p14) 20-minute walk at a comfortable pace	daily stretch (p14) 20-minute walk at a comfortable pace	daily stretch (p14) 20-minute walk at a comfortable pace
daily stretch (p14) 20-minute walk at a comfortable pace	daily stretch (p14) 20-minute walk at a comfortable pace	daily stretch (p14), 20-minute cardio, supine hamstring stretch, rainbows 5x, glute/piriformis stretch, forward/backward arm arc 5x, Cat into Cow 5x	daily stretch (p14) 20-minute walk at a comfortable pace
daily stretch (p14) 20-minute walk at a comfortable pace	daily stretch (p14) 20-minute walk at a comfortable pace	daily stretch (p14) supine hamstring stretch, rainbows 5x, glute/piriformis stretch, forward/backward arm arc 5x, Cat into Cow 5x, seated hamstring stretch, glute stretch, chest stretch arms in front, arms behind, repeat with straight arms above head	daily stretch (p14) 20-minute walk at a comfortable pace
daily stretch (p14) 20-minute walk, 20–30 minutes of running, cycling, swimming, or rowing at a steady pace	rest day daily stretch (p14) 20-minute walk.	daily stretch (p14) supine hamstring stretch, rainbows 5x, glute/piriformis stretch, forward/backward arm arc 5x, Cat into Cow 5x, seated hamstring stretch, glute stretch, chest stretch arms in front, arms behind, repeat with straight arms above head	daily stretch (p14) 20-minute walk, 20–30 minutes of running, cycling, swimming, or rowing at a steady pace

1

starter level 1 continued

The second half of this schedule increases the cardiovascular intensity and the pace of the daily 20-minute walk. In addition we will introduce core stability identification and exercises (see pages 26–27).

WEEK	MONDAY	TUESDAY	WEDNESDAY
5	daily stretch (p14), 20-minute walk, supine hamstring stretch, rainbows 5x, glute/piriformis stretch, forward/backward arm arc 5x, Cat into Cow 5x, seated hamstring stretch, glute stretch, chest stretch arms in front, behind, repeat straight above head	daily stretch (p14), 20-minute walk, 20–30 minutes of cardio at a steady pace	daily stretch (p14), 20-minute walk, supine hamstring stretch, rainbows 5x, glute/piriformis stretch, forward/backward arm arc 5x, Cat into Cow 5x, seated hamstring stretch, glute stretch, chest stretch arms in front, arms behind, repeat with straight arms above head
6	daily stretch (p14), faster 20-minute walk, core stability exercise 1, supine hamstring stretch, rainbows 5x, glute/piriformis stretch, forward/ backward arm arc 5x, Cat into Cow 5x, seated hamstring stretch, glute stretch, chest stretch arms in front, arms behind, and arms above head	daily stretch (p14), faster 20-minute walk, core stability exercise 1, 20–30 minutes of cardio with 3 x 3-minute intervals of brisk pace.	daily stretch (p14), faster 20-minute walk, core stability exercise 1, supine hamstring stretch, rainbows 5x, glute/piriformis stretch, forward/backward arm arc 5x, Cat into Cow 5x, seated hamstring stretch, glute stretch, chest stretch arms in front, arms behind, and arms above head
7	daily stretch (p14), core stability exercises 1 and 2, supine hamstring stretch, rainbows 5x, glute/piriformis stretch, forward/backward arm arc 5x, Cat into Cow 5x, seated hamstring stretch, glute stretch, chest stretch arms in front, arms behind, and arms above head	daily stretch (p14) and faster 20-minute walk, core stability exercise 1, 20–30 minutes of cardio with 3 x 3-minute intervals of brisk pace	daily stretch (p14), 20-minute walk, core stability exercises 1 and 2, supine hamstring stretch, rainbows 5x, glute/piriformis stretch, forward/backward arm arc 5x, Cat into Cow 5x, seated hamstring stretch, glute stretch, chest stretch arms in front, arms behind, and arms above head
8	daily stretch (p14), 20-minute walk, core stability exercises 1, 2 and 3, supine hamstring stretch, rainbows 5x, glute/piriformis stretch, forward/backward arm arc 5x, Cat into Cow 5x, seated hamstring stretch, glute stretch, chest stretch arms in front, arms behind, repeat with arms above head	daily stretch (p14) and faster 20-minute walk, core stability exercises 1, 2, and 3, 20–30 minutes of cardio with 3 x 3-minute intervals of brisk pace	daily stretch (p14), 20-minute walk, core stability exercises 1, 2 and 3, supine hamstring stretch, rainbows 5x, glute/piriformis stretch, forward/backward arm arc 5x, Cat into Cow 5x, seated hamstring stretch, glute stretch, chest stretch arms in front, arms behind, repeat with arms above head

WEEK 7—HOW IS IT GOING?

You should now be well into the routine of your daily schedules and feeling ready to progress. In weeks 7, 8, we introduce some core stability exercises; these will become essential to build strength in your abdomen to progress to more challenging stretch routines. Also by the end of week 8 you should be comfortable with 30 minutes steady cardio exercise, and be ready to push up the intensity. So move on to level 2. Or if you prefer, repeat weeks 4 to 8 until you feel ready to move up to level 3.

THURSDAY	FRIDAY	SATURDAY	SUNDAY
daily stretch (p14), 20-minute walk, 20–30 minutes of cardio at a steady pace	rest day daily stretch (p14) and 20-minute walk	daily stretch (p14), 20-minute walk, supine hamstring stretch, rainbows 5x, glute/piriformis stretch, forward /backward arm arc 5x, Cat into Cow 5x, seated hamstring stretch, glute stretch, chest stretch arms in front, arms behind, repeat with straight arms above head	daily stretch (p14), 20-minute walk, 20–30 minutes of cardio at a steady pace
daily stretch (p14) and faster 20-minute walk, core stability exercise 1, 20–30 minutes of cardio with 3x 3-minute intervals of brisk pace	rest day daily stretch (p14) and 20-minute walk	daily stretch (p14), faster 20-minute walk, core stability exercise 1, supine hamstring stretch, rainbows 5x, glute/piriformis stretch, forward/backward arm arc 5x, Cat into Cow 5x, seated hamstring stretch, glute stretch, chest stretch arms in front, arms behind, and arms above head	daily stretch (p14), faster 20-minute walk, core stability exercise 1, 20–30 minutes of cardio with 3 x 3-minute intervals of brisk pace
daily stretch (p14) and faster 20-minute walk, core stability exercise 1, 20–30 minutes of cardio with 3x 3-minute intervals of brisk pace	rest day daily stretch (p14) and 20-minute walk	daily stretch (p14), core stability exercises 1 and 2, supine hamstring stretch, rainbows 5x, glute/piriformis stretch, forward /backward arm arc 5x, Cat into Cow 5x, seated hamstring stretch, glute stretch, chest stretch arms in front, arms behind, repeat with arms above head	daily stretch (p14), faster 20-minute walk, core stability exercise 1, 20–30 minutes of cardio with 3 x 3-minute intervals of brisk pace
daily stretch (p14) and faster 20-minute walk, core stability exercise 1, 20–30 minutes of cardio with 3x 3-minute intervals of brisk pace	rest day daily stretch (p14) and 20-minute walk	daily stretch (p14), 20-minute walk, core stability exercises 1, 2, and 3 supine hamstring stretch, rainbows 5x, glute/piriformis stretch, forward/backward arm arc 5x, Cat into Cow 5x, seated hamstring stretch, glute stretch, chest stretch arms in front, arms behind, repeat with arms above head	daily stretch (p14), faster 20-minute walk, core stability exercise 1, 20–30 minutes of cardio with 3 x 3-minute intervals of brisk pace

starter level 2

If you are already fairly fit and have had some recent activity, this schedule should be a good starting point. The aim of this schedule is to return to daily progressive activity with confidence and to reduce aches and pains.

WEEK	MONDAY	TUESDAY	WEDNESDAY
1	daily stretch (p14), 20-minute walk	daily stretch (p14), 20-minute walk	daily stretch (p14), 20-minute walk
2	daily stretch (p14), 20-minute walk, supine hamstring stretch, rainbows 5x, glute/piriformis stretch, forward /backward arm arc 5x, Cat into Cow 5x, seated hamstring stretch, glute stretch, chest stretch arms in front, arms behind, repeat with arms above head	daily stretch (p14), 20-minute walk	daily stretch (p14), 20-minute walk, supine hamstring stretch, rainbows 5x, glute/piriformis stretch, forward /backward arm arc 5x, Cat into Cow 5x, seated hamstring stretch, glute stretch, chest stretch arms in front, arms behind, repeat with arms above head
3	daily stretch (p14), 20-minute walk, supine hamstring stretch, rainbows 5x, glute/piriformis stretch, forward /backward arm arc 5x, Cat into Cow 5x, seated hamstring stretch, glute stretch, chest stretch arms in front, arms behind, repeat with arms above head	daily stretch (p14) and 20-minute walk, 20–30 minutes of cardio at a steady pace	daily stretch (p14), 20-minute walk, supine hamstring stretch, rainbows 5x, glute/piriformis stretch, forward /backward arm arc 5x, Cat into Cow 5x, seated hamstring stretch, glute stretch, chest stretch arms in front, arms behind, repeat with arms above head
4	daily stretch (p14), 20-minute walk, core stability exercise 1, supine hamstring stretch, rainbows 5x, glute/piriformis stretch, forward/backward arm arc 5x, Cat into Cow 5x, seated hamstring stretch, glute stretch, chest stretch arms in front, arms behind, and arms above head.	daily stretch (p14) and 20-minute walk, 20–30 minutes of cardio at a steady pace	daily stretch (p14), 20-minute walk, core stability exercise 1, supine hamstring stretch, rainbows 5x, glute/piriformis stretch, forward/ backward arm arc 5x, Cat into Cow 5x, seated hamstring stretch, glute stretch, chest stretch arms in front, arms behind, and arms above head

WEEK 4—HOW'S IT GOING?

Be sure to take your time. If you are becoming frequently tired, or if you have persistent aches and pains, ease off the pace and do not hesitate to replace a long or hard run with a shorter or easier one.

THURSDAY	FRIDAY	SATURDAY	SUNDAY
daily stretch (p14), 20-minute walk	daily stretch (p14), 20-minute walk	daily stretch (p14), 20-minute walk	daily stretch (p14), 20-minute walk
daily stretch (p14) 20-minute walk.	daily stretch (p14), 30-minute walk	daily stretch (p14), 30-minute walk, supine hamstring stretch, rainbows 5x, glute/piriformis stretch, forward/backward arm arc 5x, Cat into Cow 5x, seated hamstring stretch, glute stretch, chest stretch arms in front, arms behind, repeat with arms above head	daily stretch (p14), 20-minute walk
daily stretch (p14) and 20-minute walk, 20–30 minutes of cardio at a steady pace	rest day daily stretch (p14), 30–minute walk	daily stretch (p14), 20-minute walk, supine hamstring stretch, rainbows 5x, glute/piriformis stretch, forward/backward arm arc 5x, Cat into Cow 5x, seated hamstring stretch, glute stretch, chest stretch arms in front, arms behind, repeat with arms above head	daily stretch (p14), 20-minute walk
daily stretch (p14), 20-minute walk, core stability exercise 1, 20–30 minutes of cardio at a steady pace	daily stretch (p14), 20-minute walk	daily stretch (p14), 20-minute walk, core stability exercise 1, supine hamstring stretch, rainbows 5x, glute/piriformis stretch, forward/backward arm arc 5x, Cat into Cow 5x, seated hamstring stretch, glute stretch, chest stretch arms in front, arms behind, repeat with arms above head	daily stretch (p14), 20-minute walk, core stability exercise 1, 20–30 minutes of cardio at a steady pace

2

starter level 2 continued

WEEK	MONDAY	TUESDAY	WEDNESDAY
5	daily stretch (p14), 20-minute walk, core stability exercise 1, supine hamstring stretch, rainbows 5x, glute/piriformis stretch, forward/backward arm arc 5x, Cat into Cow 5x, hamstring stretch, glute stretch, chest stretch arms in front, arms behind, and arms above head, cobra, lying pelvic tilts 5x, chalk circles 3x, seated adductor stretch, sitting twist stretch, wall push-ups 2x5 reps, core exercise 2	daily stretch (p14), 20-minute walk, core stability exercise 1, 20–30 minutes of cardio at a steady pace	daily stretch (p14), 20-minute walk, core stability exercise 1, supine hamstring stretch, rainbows 5x, glute/piriformis stretch, forward/backward arm arc 5x, Cat into Cow 5x, hamstring stretch, glute stretch, chest stretch arms in front, arms behind, and arms above head, cobra, lying pelvic tilts 5x, chalk circles 3x, seated adductor stretch, sitting twist stretch, wall push-ups 2x5 reps, core exercise 2
6	daily stretch(p14), 20-minute walk, core stability exercises 1 and 3, supine hamstring stretch, rainbows 5x, glute/piriformis stretch, forward /backward arm arc 5x, Cat into Cow 5x, hamstring stretch, glute stretch, chest stretch arms in front, arms behind, and arms above head, cobra, lying pelvic tilts 5x, chalk circles 3x, seated adductor stretch, sitting twist stretch, wall push-ups 2x5 reps, core exercise 2	daily stretch (p14), 20-minute walk, core stability exercise 1, 20–30 minutes of cardio at a steady pace	daily stretch (p14), 20-minute walk, core stability exercises 1 and 3, supine hamstring stretch, rainbows 5x, glute/piriformis stretch, forward/ backward arm arc 5x, Cat into Cow 5x, hamstring stretch, glute stretch, chest stretch arms in front, arms behind, and arms above head, cobra, lying pelvic tilts 5x, chalk circles 3x, seated adductor stretch, sitting twist stretch, wall push-ups 2x5 reps, core exercise 2
7	daily stretch and 20 minute walk, core stability exercises 1 and 3, supine hamstring stretch, rainbows 5x, glute/piriformis stretch, forward /backward arm arc 5x, Cat into Cow 5x, hamstring stretch, glute stretch, chest stretch arms in front, arms behind, and arms above head, cobra, lying pelvic tilts 5x, chalk circles 3x, seated adductor stretch, sitting twist stretch, wall push-ups 2x5 reps, core exercise 2	daily stretch (p14), 20-minute walk, core stability exercise 1, 20–30 minutes of cardio at a steady pace	daily stretch (p14), 20-minute walk, core stability exercises 1 and 3, supine hamstring stretch, rainbows 5x, glute/piriformis stretch, forward /backward arm arc 5x, Cat into Cow 5x, hamstring stretch, glute stretch, chest stretch arms in front, arms behind, and arms above head, cobra, lying pelvic tilts 5x, chalk circles 3x, seated adductor stretch, sitting twist stretch, wall push-ups 2x5 reps, core exercise 2
8	**REPEAT WEEK 7**	**REPEAT WEEK 7**	**REPEAT WEEK 7**

THURSDAY	FRIDAY	SATURDAY	SUNDAY
daily stretch (p14), 20-minute walk, core stability exercise 1, 20–30 minutes of cardio at a steady pace	rest day daily stretch (p14), 20-minute walk	daily stretch (p14), 20-minute walk, core stability exercise 1, supine hamstring stretch, rainbows 5x, glute/piriformis stretch, forward/backward arm arc 5x, Cat into Cow 5x, hamstring stretch, glute stretch, chest stretch arms in front, arms behind, and arms above head, cobra, lying pelvic tilts 5x, chalk circles 3x, seated adductor stretch, sitting twist stretch, wall push-ups 2x5 reps, core exercise 2	daily stretch (p14), 20-minute walk, core stability exercise 1, 20–30 minutes of cardio at a steady pace
daily stretch (p14), 20-minute walk, core stability exercise 1, 20–30 minutes of cardio at a steady pace	rest day daily stretch (p14), 20-minute walk	daily stretch (p14), 20-minute walk, core stability exercises 1 and 3, supine hamstring stretch, rainbows x5, glute/piriformis stretch, forward /backward arm arc 5x, Cat into Cow 5x, hamstring stretch, glute stretch, chest stretch arms in front, arms behind, and arms above head, cobra, lying pelvic tilts 5x, chalk circles 3x, seated adductor stretch, sitting twist stretch, wall push-ups 2x5 reps, core exercise 2	daily stretch (p14) 20-minute walk, core stability exercise 1, 20–30 minutes of cardio at a steady pace
daily stretch (p14), 20-minute walk, core stability exercise 1, 20–30 minutes of cardio at a steady pace	rest day daily stretch (p14), 20-minute walk	daily stretch (p14), 20-minute walk, core stability exercises 1 and 3, supine hamstring stretch, rainbows 5x, glute/piriformis stretch, forward /backward arm arc 5x, Cat into Cow 5x, hamstring stretch, glute stretch, chest stretch arms in front, arms behind, and arms above head, cobra, lying pelvic tilts 5x, chalk circles 3x, seated adductor stretch, sitting twist stretch, wall push-ups 2x5 reps, core exercise 2	daily stretch (p14), 20-minute walk, core stability exercise 1, 20–30 minutes of cardio at a steady pace
REPEAT WEEK 7		**REPEAT WEEK 7**	**REPEAT WEEK 7**

intermediate level 1

For people who are generally active but not in regular exercise or sports. The aim of this schedule is to focus activity and progression and to reduce aches and pains.

WEEK	MONDAY	TUESDAY	WEDNESDAY
1	daily stretch (p14), 20-minute walk	daily stretch (p14), 20-minute walk	daily stretch (p14), 20-minute walk
2	daily stretch (p14), 20-minute walk, supine hamstring stretch, rainbows 5x, glute/piriformis stretch, forward/backward arm arc 5x, Cat into Cow 5x, hamstring stretch, glute stretch, chest stretch arms in front, arms behind, and arms above head, wall push-ups 5x reps	daily stretch (p14), 20-minute walk, 20–30 minutes of cardio at a steady pace	daily stretch (p14), 20-minute walk, supine hamstring stretch, rainbows 5x, glute/piriformis stretch, forward /backward arm arc 5x, Cat into Cow 5x, hamstring stretch, glute stretch, chest stretch arms in front, arms behind, and arms above head, wall push-ups 5x reps
3	daily stretch(p14), 20-minute walk, core stability exercise 1, supine hamstring stretch, rainbows 5x, glute/piriformis stretch, forward/backward arm arc 5x, Cat into Cow 5x, hamstring stretch, glute stretch, chest stretch arms in front, arms behind, and arms above head, wall push-ups 5x	daily stretch (p14), 20-minute walk, core stability exercise 1, 20–30 minutes of cardio at a steady pace	daily stretch (p14), 20-minute walk, core stability exercise 1, supine hamstring stretch, rainbows 5x, glute/piriformis stretch, forward/backward arm arc 5x, Cat into Cow 5x, hamstring stretch, glute stretch, chest stretch arms in front, arms behind, and arms above head, wall push-ups 5x
4	daily stretch(p14), 20-minute walk, core stability exercises 1 and 2, supine hamstring stretch, rainbows 5x, glute/piriformis stretch, forward/backward arm arc 5x, Cat into Cow 5x, hamstring stretch, glute stretch, chest stretch arms in front, arms behind, and arms above head, wall push-ups 10x	daily stretch (p14), 20-minute walk, core stability exercise 1, 20–30 minutes of cardio with 3 x 3-minute intervals of brisk pace	daily stretch (p14), 20-minute walk, core stability exercises 1 and 2, supine hamstring stretch, rainbows 5x, glute/piriformis stretch, forward/ backward arm arc 5x, Cat into Cow 5x, hamstring stretch, glute stretch, chest stretch arms in front, arms behind, and arms above head, wall push-ups 10x reps

WEEK 4—HOW'S IT GOING?

Be sure to take your time. If you are becoming frequently tired, or if you have persistent aches and pains, do not hesitate to reduce the pace of your cardio workouts, and cut out the brisk 3-minute intervals. If it feels comfortable, repeat week 4, or if you wish, repeat week 3 without the intervals.

THURSDAY	FRIDAY	SATURDAY	SUNDAY
daily stretch (p14), 20-minute walk	daily stretch (p14), 20-minute walk	daily stretch (p14), 20-minute walk	daily stretch (p14), 20-minute walk
daily stretch (p14), 20-minute walk, 20–30 minutes of cardio at a steady pace	rest day daily stretch (p14), 20-minute walk	daily stretch (p14), 20-minute walk, supine hamstring stretch, rainbows 5x, glute/piriformis stretch, forward/backward arm arc 5x, Cat into Cow 5x, hamstring stretch, glute stretch, chest stretch arms in front, arms behind, and arms above head, wall push-ups 5x reps	daily stretch (p14), 20-minute walk, 20–30 minutes of cardio at a steady pace
daily stretch (p14), 20-minute walk, core stability exercise 1, 20–30 minutes of cardio at a steady pace	rest day daily stretch (p14), 20-minute walk	daily stretch (p14), 20-minute walk, core stability exercise 1, supine hamstring stretch, rainbows 5x, glute/piriformis stretch, forward/backward arm arc 5x, Cat into Cow 5x, hamstring stretch, glute stretch, chest stretch arms in front, arms behind, and arms above head, wall push-ups 5x	daily stretch (p14), 20-minute walk, core stability exercise 1, 20–30 minutes of cardio at a steady pace
daily stretch (p14), 20-minute walk, core stability exercise 1, 20–30 minutes of cardio with 3 x 3-minute intervals of brisk pace	rest day daily stretch (p14), 20-minute walk	daily stretch (p14), 20-minute walk, core stability exercise 1 and 2, supine hamstring stretch, rainbows 5x, glute/piriformis stretch, forward/backward arm arc 5x, Cat into Cow 5x, hamstring stretch, glute stretch, chest stretch arms in front, arms behind, and arms above head, wall push-ups 10x reps	daily stretch (p14), 20-minute walk, core stability exercise 1, 20–30 minutes of cardio with 3x 3-minute intervals of brisk pace

3

intermediate level 1 continued

WEEK	MONDAY	TUESDAY	WEDNESDAY
5	daily stretch (p14), 20-minute walk, core stability exercises 1, 2, and 3, supine hamstring stretch, rainbows x5, glute/piriformis stretch, forward/backward arm arc 5x, Cat into Cow 5x, hamstring stretch, glute stretch, chest stretch arms in front, arms behind, and arms above head, cobra, box push-ups 5x, pelvic tilt, curl up to bridge 5x, chalk circles 3x, sitting adductor stretch, seated twist, standing crucifix, over/under hand clasp	daily stretch (p14), 20-minute walk, core stability exercise 1 and 3, 30–40 minutes cardio with 3 x 3-minute intervals of brisk pace	daily stretch (p14), 20-minute walk, core stability exercises 1, 2, and 3, supine hamstring stretch, rainbows 5x, glute /piriformis stretch, forward/backward arm arc 5x, Cat into Cow 5x, hamstring stretch, glute stretch, chest stretch arms in front, arms behind, and arms above head, cobra, box push-ups 5x, pelvic tilt, curl up to bridge 5x, chalk circles 3x, sitting adductor stretch, seated twist, standing crucifix, over/under hand clasp
6	daily stretch (p14), 20-minute walk, core stability exercises 1, 2, and 3, supine hamstring stretch, rainbows 5x, glute/piriformis stretch, forward/backward arm arc 5x, Cat into Cow 5x, hamstring stretch, glute stretch, chest stretch arms in front, arms behind, and arms above head, cobra, box push-ups 5x, pelvic tilt, curl up to bridge 5x, chalk circles 3x, sitting adductor stretch, seated twist, standing crucifix, over/under hand clasp	daily stretch (p14), 20-minute walk, core stability exercise 1 and 3, 30–40 minutes cardio with 3 x 3-minute intervals of brisk pace	daily stretch (p14), 20-minute walk, core stability exercises 1, 2, and 3, supine hamstring stretch, rainbows 5x, glute /piriformis stretch, forward/backward arm arc 5x, Cat into Cow 5x, hamstring stretch, glute stretch, chest stretch arms in front, arms behind, and arms above head, cobra, box push-ups 5x, pelvic tilt, curl up to bridge 5x, chalk circles 3x, sitting adductor stretch, seated twist, standing crucifix, over/under hand clasp
7	daily stretch (p14), 20-minute walk, core stability exercises 1, 2, 3, and 4, supine hamstring, rainbows 5x, glute/piriformis, forward/backward arm arc 5x, Cat into Cow 5x, seated hamstring, glute; chest stretch arms in front, arms behind, and arms above head, cobra, box push-ups 5x, pelvic tilt, curl up to bridge 5x, chalk circles 3x, seated adductor, seated twist, standing crucifix, over/under hand clasp, chair supp. squat and lunge 5x	daily stretch (p14), 20-minute walk, core stability exercise 1 and 3, 30–40 minutes cardio with 3 x 3-minute intervals of brisk pace	daily stretch (p14), 20-minute walk, core stability exercises 1, 2, 3, and 4, supine hamstring, rainbows 5x, glute/piriformis, forward/backward arm arc 5x, Cat into Cow 5x, hamstring stretch, glute, chest arms in front, arms behind, and arms above head, cobra, box push-ups 5x, pelvic tilt, curl up to bridge 5x, chalk circles 3x, sitting adductor, seated twist, standing crucifix, over/under hand clasp, chair supp. squat and lunge 5x
8	SEE PANEL OPPOSITE TOP		

WEEK 8—STEP IT UP

Now is the time to really start building up the exercise. Repeat week 7 and add one legged bridge, seated adductors, 90 degree squat, and lunge. Increase cardio work to 45 minutes with 6x 2-minute brisk intervals. You may be getting bored with cardio so try to vary what you do; try a mix of walking, cycling, running, or even try an exercise class at the gym.

THURSDAY	FRIDAY	SATURDAY	SUNDAY
daily stretch (p14), 20-minute walk, core stability exercises 1 and 3, 20–30 minutes cardio with 3x 3-minute intervals of brisk pace	rest day daily stretch (p14), 20-minute walk	daily stretch (p14), 20-minute walk, core stability exercises 1,2, and 3, supine hamstring stretch, rainbows 5x, glute/piriformis stretch, forward /backward arm arc 5x, Cat into Cow 5x, hamstring stretch, glute stretch, chest stretch arms in front, arms behind, and arms above head, cobra, box push-ups 5x, pelvic tilt, curl up to bridge 5x, chalk circles 3x, sitting adductor stretch, seated twist, standing crucifix, over/under hand clasp	daily stretch (p14), 20-minute walk, core stability exercises 1 and 3, 20–30 minutes cardio with 3x 3-minute intervals of brisk pace
daily stretch (p14), 20-minute walk, core stability exercises 1 and 3, 30–40 minutes cardio with 3x 3-minute intervals of brisk pace	rest day daily stretch (p14), 20-minute walk	daily stretch (p14), 20-minute walk, core stability exercises 1,2, and 3, supine hamstring stretch, rainbows 5x, glute/piriformis stretch, forward /backward arm arc 5x, Cat into Cow 5x, hamstring stretch, glute stretch, chest stretch arms in front, arms behind, and arms above head, cobra, box push-ups 5x, pelvic tilt, curl up to bridge 5x, chalk circles 3x, sitting adductor stretch, seated twist, standing crucifix, over/under hand clasp	daily stretch (p14), 20-minute walk, core stability exercises 1 and 3, 30–40 minutes cardio with 3x 3-minute intervals of brisk pace
daily stretch (p14), 20-minute walk, core stability exercises 1 and 3, 30–40 minutes cardio with 3x 3 minute intervals of brisk pace	rest day daily stretch (p14), 20-minute walk	daily stretch (p14), 20-minute walk, core stability exercises 1, 2, 3, and 4, supine hamstring, rainbows 5x, glute/piriformis, forward/backward arm arc 5x, Cat into Cow 5x, hamstring stretch, glute, chest arms in front, arms behind, and arms above head, cobra, box push-ups 5x, pelvic tilt, curl up to bridge 5x, chalk circles 3x, sitting adductor, seated twist, standing crucifix, over/under hand clasp, chair supp. squat and lunge 5x	daily stretch (p14), 20-minute walk, core stability exercises 1 and 3, 30–40 minutes cardio with 3x 3-minute intervals of brisk pace

If you can keep this schedule up for another 3 weeks you can no longer say that you are just generally active; you have joined the regulars!

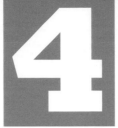

intermediate level 2

For people who are in regular exercise or sports maybe once or twice a week, but want to stretch more to help build on their fitness.

WEEK	MONDAY	TUESDAY	WEDNESDAY	
1	daily stretch (p15), 20-minute walk	daily stretch (p15), 20-minute walk	daily stretch (p15), 20-minute walk	
2	daily stretch (p15), 20-minute walk, core stability exercise 1, supine hamstring stretch, rainbows 5x, glute/piriformis stretch, hamstring stretch, glute stretch, chest stretch arms in front, arms behind, and arms above head, wall push-ups 10x reps.	daily stretch, 20-minute walk, core stability exercise 1, 40 minutes cardio with 6x 2-minute intervals of brisk pace	daily stretch (p15), 20-minute walk, core stability exercise 1, supine hamstring stretch, rainbows 5x, glute/piriformis stretch, hamstring stretch, glute stretch, chest stretch arms in front, arms behind, and arms above head, wall push-ups 10x reps	
3	daily stretch (p15), 20-minute walk, core stability exercises 1, 2, and 3, supine hamstring stretch, rainbows 5x, glute/piriformis stretch, hamstring stretch, glute stretch, chest stretch arms in front, arms behind, and arms above head, wall push-ups 10x reps	daily stretch, 20-minute walk, core stability exercise 1, 40 minutes cardio with 6x 2-minute intervals of brisk pace	daily stretch (p15), 20-minute walk, core stability exercises 1, 2, and 3, supine hamstring stretch, rainbows 5x, glute/piriformis stretch, hamstring stretch, glute stretch, chest stretch arms in front, arms behind, and arms above head, wall push-ups 10x reps	
4	daily stretch (p15), 20-minute walk, core stability exercises 1, 2, and 3, supine hamstring stretch, rainbows 5x, glute/piriformis stretch, hamstring stretch, glute stretch, chest stretch arms in front, arms behind, and arms above head, wall push-ups x10 reps, cobra, box push-ups 5x, pelvic tilt and curl up to bridge 5x, sitting adductor stretch, sitting twist, squats, heels down, knees to 90 5x, standing quads stretch, standing hams stretch, lunge 5x, standing crucifix 5x, over/under hand clasp	daily stretch, 20-minute walk, core stability exercise 1, 40 minutes cardio with 6x 2-minute intervals of brisk pace	daily stretch (p15), 20-minute walk, core stability exercises 1, 2, and 3, supine hamstring stretch, rainbows 5x, glute/piriformis stretch, hamstring stretch, glute stretch, chest stretch arms in front, arms behind, and arms above head, wall push-ups 10x reps, cobra, box push-ups 5x, pelvic tilt and curl up to bridge 5x, sitting adductor stretch, sitting twist, squats, heels down, knees to 90 5x, standing quads stretch, standing hams stretch, lunge 5x, standing crucifix 5x, over/under hand clasp	

IF YOU ARE DOING REGULAR EXERCISE

Just do one of the stretching sessions on gym or sports days, and if you are already doing some cardiovascular exercise, you just need to total three sessions of at least 20 minutes.
If your current program doesn't include cardiovascular work, you will need to bring up your level of cardiovascular fitness to the ability to do 20 minutes at an easy pace without stopping.

THURSDAY	FRIDAY	SATURDAY	SUNDAY
daily stretch (p15), 20-minute walk	daily stretch (p15), 20-minute walk	daily stretch (p15), 20-minute walk	daily stretch (p15), 20-minute walk
daily stretch, 20-minute walk, core stability exercise 1, 40 minutes cardio with 6x 2-minute intervals of brisk pace	daily stretch (p15), 20-minute walk, core stability exercise 1, supine hamstring stretch, rainbows 5x, glute/piriformis stretch, hamstring stretch, glute stretch, chest stretch arms in front, arms behind, and arms above head, wall push-ups 10x reps	rest day daily stretch (p15), 20-minute walk	daily stretch (p15), 20-minute walk, core stability exercise 1, 40 minutes cardio with 6x 2-minute intervals of brisk pace
daily stretch, 20-minute walk, core stability exercise 1 and 3, 40 minutes cardio with 6x 2-minute intervals of brisk pace	daily stretch (p15), 20-minute walk, core stability exercises 1, 2, and 3, supine hamstring stretch, rainbows 5x, glute/piriformis stretch, hamstring stretch, glute stretch, chest stretch arms in front, arms behind, and arms above head, wall push-ups 10x reps	rest day daily stretch (p15), 20-minute walk	daily stretch (p15), 20-minute walk, core stability exercises 1 and 3, 40 minutes cardio with 6x 2-minute intervals of brisk pace
daily stretch, 20-minute walk, core stability exercises 1 and 3, 40 minutes cardio with 6x 2-minute intervals of brisk pace	daily stretch(p15), 20-minute walk, core stability exercises 1, 2, and 3, supine hamstring stretch, rainbows 5x, glute/piriformis stretch, hamstring stretch, glute stretch, chest stretch arms in front, arms behind, and arms above head, wall push-ups 10x reps, cobra, box push-ups 5x, pelvic tilt and curl up to bridge 5x, sitting adductor stretch, sitting twist, squats, heels down, knees to 90 5x, standing quads stretch, standing hams stretch, lunge 5x, standing crucifix 5x, over/under hand clasp	rest day daily stretch (p15), 20-minute walk	daily stretch (p15), 20-minute walk, core stability exercises 1 and 3, 40 minutes cardio with 6x 2-minute intervals of brisk pace

4

intermediate level 2 continued

WEEK	MONDAY	TUESDAY	WEDNESDAY
5	daily stretch (p15), 20-minute walk, core stability exercises 1, 2, 3, and 4, supine hamstring stretch, rainbows 5x, glute/piriformis stretch, hamstring stretch, glute stretch, chest stretch arms in front, arms behind, and arms above head, wall push-ups 10x reps, cobra, box push-ups 5x, pelvic tilt and curl up to bridge 5x, sitting adductor stretch, sitting twist, squats, heels down, knees to 90 5x, standing quads stretch, standing hams stretch, lunge 5x, standing crucifix 5x, over/under hand clasp	daily stretch (p15), 20-minute walk, core stability exercises 1 and 3, 40 minutes cardio with 6x 2-minute intervals of brisk pace	daily stretch (p15), 20-minute walk, core stability exercises 1, 2, 3, and 4, supine hamstring stretch, rainbows 5x, glute/piriformis stretch, hamstring stretch, glute stretch, chest stretch arms in front, arms behind, and arms above head, wall push-ups 10x reps, cobra, box push-ups 5x, pelvic tilt and curl up to bridge 5x, sitting adductor stretch, sitting twist, squats, heels down, knees to 90 5x, standing quads stretch, standing hams stretch, lunge 5x, standing crucifix 5x, over/under hand clasp
6	daily stretch (p15), 20-minute walk, core stability exercises 1, 2, 3, and 4, supine hamstring stretch, rainbows 5x, glute/piriformis stretch, hamstring stretch, glute stretch, chest stretch arms in front, arms behind, and arms above head, wall push-ups 10x reps, cobra, box push-ups 5x, pelvic tilt and curl up to bridge 5x, sitting adductor stretch, sitting twist, squats, heels down, knees to 90 5x, standing quads stretch, standing hams stretch, lunge 5x, standing crucifix 5x, over/under hand clasp	daily stretch (p15), 20-minute walk, core stability exercises 1 and 3, 40 minutes cardio with 6x 2-minute intervals of brisk pace	daily stretch (p15), 20-minute walk, core stability exercises 1, 2, 3, and 4, supine hamstring stretch, rainbows 5x, glute/piriformis stretch, hamstring stretch, glute stretch, chest stretch arms in front, arms behind, and arms above head, wall push-ups 10x reps, cobra, box push-ups 5x, pelvic tilt and curl up to bridge 5x, sitting adductor stretch, sitting twist, squats, heels down, knees to 90 5x, standing quads stretch, standing hams stretch, lunge 5x, standing crucifix 5x, over/under hand clasp
7	daily stretch (p15), 20-minute walk, core stability exercises 1, 2, 3, and 4, supine hamstring stretch, rainbows 5x, glute/piriformis stretch, hamstring stretch, glute stretch, chest stretch arms in front, arms behind, and arms above head, wall push-ups 10x reps, cobra, box push-ups 5x, pelvic tilt and curl up to bridge 5x, sitting adductor stretch, sitting twist, squats, heels down, knees to 90 5x, standing quads stretch, standing hams stretch, lunge 5x, standing crucifix 5x, over/under hand clasp	daily stretch (p15), 20-minute walk, core stability exercises 1 and 3, 40 minutes cardio with 6x 2-minute intervals of brisk pace	daily stretch (p15), 20-minute walk, core stability exercises 1, 2, 3, and 4, supine hamstring stretch, rainbows 5x, glute/piriformis stretch, hamstring stretch, glute stretch, chest stretch arms in front, arms behind, and arms above head, wall push-ups 10x reps, cobra, box push-ups 5x, pelvic tilt and curl up to bridge 5x, sitting adductor stretch, sitting twist, squats, heels down, knees to 90 5x, standing quads stretch, standing hams stretch, lunge 5x, standing crucifix 5x, over/under hand clasp
8	**REPEAT WEEK 7**	**INCREASE CARDIO TO 45 MINUTES AND DO 8X 2-MINUTE INTERVALS OF BRISK PACE.**	

THURSDAY	FRIDAY	SATURDAY	SUNDAY
daily stretch, 20-minute walk, core stability exercises 1 and 3, 40 minutes cardio with 6x 2-minute intervals of brisk pace	daily stretch (p15), 20-minute walk, core stability exercises 1, 2, 3, and 4, supine hamstring stretch, rainbows 5x, glute/piriformis stretch, hamstring stretch, glute stretch, chest stretch arms in front, arms behind, and arms above head, wall push-ups 10x reps, cobra, box push-ups 5x, pelvic tilt and curl up to bridge 5x, sitting adductor stretch, sitting twist, squats, heels down, knees to 90 5x, standing quads stretch, standing hams stretch, lunge 5x, standing crucifix 5x, over/under hand clasp	rest day daily stretch (p15), 20-minute walk	daily stretch (p15), 20-minute walk, core stability exercises 1 and 3, 40 minutes cardio with 6x 2-minute intervals of brisk pace
daily stretch, 20-minute walk, core stability exercises 1 and 3, 40 minutes cardio with 6x 2-minute intervals of brisk pace	daily stretch (p15), 20-minute walk, core stability exercises 1, 2, 3, and 4, supine hamstring stretch, rainbows 5x, glute/piriformis stretch, hamstring stretch, glute stretch, chest stretch arms in front, arms behind, and arms above head, wall push-ups 10x reps, cobra, box push-ups 5x, pelvic tilt and curl up to bridge 5x, sitting adductor stretch, sitting twist, squats, heels down, knees to 90 5x, standing quads stretch, standing hams stretch, lunge 5x, standing crucifix 5x, over/under hand clasp	rest day daily stretch (p15), 20-minute walk	daily stretch (p15), 20-minute walk, core stability exercises 1 and 3, 40 minutes cardio with 6x 2-minute intervals of brisk pace
daily stretch, 20-minute walk, core stability exercises 1 and 3, 40 minutes cardio with 6x 2-minute intervals of brisk pace	daily stretch (p15), 20-minute walk, core stability exercises 1, 2, 3, and 4, supine hamstring stretch, rainbows 5x, glute/piriformis stretch, hamstring stretch, glute stretch, chest stretch arms in front, arms behind, and arms above head, wall push-ups 10x reps, cobra, box push-ups 5x, pelvic tilt and curl up to bridge 5x, sitting adductor stretch, sitting twist, squats, heels down, knees to 90 5x, standing quads stretch, standing hams stretch, lunge 5x, standing crucifix 5x, over/under hand clasp	rest day daily stretch (p15), 20-minute walk	daily stretch (p15), 20-minute walk, core stability exercises 1 and 3, 40 minutes cardio with 6x 2-minute intervals of brisk pace

upper level 1

Now you are taking regular exercise perhaps three or four times per week and you will want to stretch more to build on your level of fitness and capitalize on all that hard work!

WEEK	MONDAY	TUESDAY	WEDNESDAY
1	daily stretch (p15), 20-minute walk, core stability exercise 1	daily stretch (p15), 20-minute walk, core stability exercise 1	daily stretch (p15), 20-minute walk, core stability exercise 1
2	daily stretch (p15), 20-minute walk, core stability identification and exercises 1, 2, and 3, hamstring stretch, rainbows 5x, glute/piriformis stretch, pelvic tilt 5x, cobra stretch, prone trunk raise 5x, push-ups 10x, seated hamstring stretch, seated glute stretch, seated twist, seated adductor stretch, chest stretch, crucifix 5x, under/over hand clasp	daily stretch (p15), 20-minute walk, core stability exercise 1, 40 minutes cardio with 2-minute intervals of brisk pace	daily stretch (p15), 20-minute walk, core stability identification and exercises 1, 2, and 3, hamstring stretch, rainbows 5x, glute/piriformis stretch, pelvic tilt 5x, cobra stretch, prone trunk raise 5x, push-ups 10x, seated hamstring stretch, seated glute stretch, seated twist, seated adductor stretch, chest stretch, crucifix 5x, under/over hand clasp
3	daily stretch (p15), 20-minute walk, core stability identification and exercise 1, 2, 3, 4, and 5, hamstring stretch, rainbows 5x, glute/piriformis stretch, pelvic tilt 5x, cobra stretch, prone trunk raise 5x, push-ups 10x, seated hamstring stretch, seated glute stretch, seated twist, seated adductor stretch, chest stretch, crucifix 5x, under/over hand clasp	daily stretch (p15), 20-minute walk, core stability exercises 1 and 3, 40 minutes cardio with 6x 2-minute intervals of brisk pace	daily stretch (p15), 20-minute walk, core stability identification and exercises 1, 2, 3, 4, and 5, hamstring stretch, rainbows 5x, glute/piriformis stretch, pelvic tilt 5x, cobra stretch, prone trunk raise 5x, push-ups x10, seated hamstring stretch, seated glute stretch, seated twist, seated adductor stretch, chest stretch, crucifix 5x, under/over hand clasp
4	daily stretch(p15), 20-minute walk, core stability 1, 2, 3, 4, and 5, ham stretch, rainbows 5x, glute/piriformis stretch, pelvic tilt 5x, cobra stretch, prone trunk raise 5x, push-ups 10x, seated ham stretch, seated glute stretch, seated twist, seated adductor stretch, chest stretch, crucifix 5x, under/over hand clasp, superman 5x, pelvic tilt up to bridge stretch 5x, seated adductor, legs apart, squats 5x, standing quad stretch, standing ham stretch, lunge 5x	daily stretch (p15), 20-minute walk, core stability exercises 1 and 3, 40 minutes cardio with 6x 2-minute intervals of brisk pace	daily stretch (p15), 20-minute walk, core stability 1, 2, 3, 4, and 5, hamstring stretch, rainbows 5x, glute/piriformis stretch, pelvic tilt 5x, cobra stretch, prone trunk raise 5x, push-ups 10x, seated ham stretch, seated glute stretch, seated twist, seated adductor stretch, chest stretch, crucifix 5x, under/over hand clasp, superman 5x, pelvic tilt up to bridge stretch 5x, seated adductor, legs apart, squats 5x, standing quad stretch, standing ham stretch, lunge 5x

WEEK 4—HOW'S IT GOING?

If you are finding the routines too much, ease back a little by reducing the cardio workouts to 30 minutes and cut out the interval training. When you feel happy and comfortable, that will indicate that you are ready to ease the cardio back up 5 minutes at a time, and slowly reintroduce the intervals.

THURSDAY	FRIDAY	SATURDAY	SUNDAY
daily stretch (p15), 20-minute walk, core stability exercise 1	daily stretch (p15), 20-minute walk, core stability exercise 1	daily stretch (p15), 20-minute walk, core stability exercise 1	daily stretch (p15), 20-minute walk, core stability exercise 1
daily stretch (p15), 20-minute walk, core stability exercise 1, 40 minutes cardio with 6x 2-minute intervals of brisk pace	daily stretch (p15), 20-minute walk, core stability identification and exercises 1, 2, and 3, hamstring stretch, rainbows 5x, glute/piriformis stretch, pelvic tilt 5x, cobra stretch, prone trunk raise 5x, push-ups 10x, seated hamstring stretch, seated glute stretch, seated twist, seated adductor stretch, chest stretch, crucifix 5x, under/over hand clasp	rest day daily stretch (p15), 20-minute walk	daily stretch (p15), 20-minute walk, core stability exercise 1, 40 minutes cardio with 6x 2-minute intervals of brisk pace
daily stretch (p15), 20-minute walk, core stability exercises 1 and 3, 40 minutes cardio with 6x 2-minute intervals of brisk pace	daily stretch (p15), 20-minute walk, core stability identification and exercises 1, 2, 3, 4, and 5, hamstring stretch, rainbows 5x, glute/piriformis stretch, pelvic tilt 5x, cobra stretch, prone trunk raise 5x, push-ups 10x, seated hamstring stretch, seated glute stretch, seated twist, seated adductor stretch, chest stretch, crucifix 5x, under/over hand clasp	rest day daily stretch (p15), 20-minute walk	daily stretch (p15), 20-minute walk, core stability exercises 1 and 3, 40 minutes cardio with 6x 2-minute intervals of brisk pace
daily stretch (p15), 20-minute walk, core stability exercises 1 and 3, 40 minutes cardio with 6x 2-minute intervals of brisk pace	daily stretch (p15), 20-minute walk, core stability 1, 2, 3, 4, and 5, ham stretch, rainbows 5x, glute/piriformis stretch, pelvic tilt 5x, cobra stretch, prone trunk raise 5x, push-ups 10x, seated ham stretch, seated glute stretch, seated twist, seated adductor stretch, chest stretch, crucifix 5x, under/over hand clasp, superman 5x, pelvic tilt up to bridge stretch 5x, seated adductor, legs apart, squats 5x, standing quad stretch, standing ham stretch, lunge 5x	rest day daily stretch (p15), 20-minute walk	daily stretch (p15), 20-minute walk, core stability exercises 1 and 3, 40 minutes cardio with 6x 2-minute intervals of brisk pace

5

upper level 1 continued

WEEK	MONDAY	TUESDAY	WEDNESDAY
5	daily stretch (p15), 20-minute walk, core stability 1, 2, 3, 4, 5, and 6, hamstring stretch, rainbows 5x, glute/piriformis stretch, pelvic tilt 5x, cobra stretch, prone trunk raise 2x5, push-ups 10x, seated ham stretch, seated glute stretch, seated twist, seated adductor stretch, chest stretch, crucifix 5x, under/over hand clasp, superman 5x, pelvic tilt up to bridge stretch 5x, seated adductor, legs apart, squats 5x, standing quad stretch, standing hamstring stretch, lunge 5x	daily stretch (p15), 20-minute walk, core stability exercise 1 and 3, 45 minutes cardio with 8x 2-minute intervals of brisk pace	daily stretch (p15), 20-minute walk, core stability 1, 2, 3, 4, 5, and 6, hamstring stretch, rainbows 5x, glute/piriformis stretch, pelvic tilt 5x, cobra stretch, prone trunk raise 2x5, push-ups 10x, seated ham stretch, seated glute stretch, seated twist, seated adductor stretch, chest stretch, crucifix 5x, under/over hand clasp, superman 5x, pelvic tilt up to bridge stretch 5x, seated adductor, legs apart, squats 5x, standing quad stretch, standing hamstring stretch, lunge 5x
6	**REPEAT WEEK 5**. Concentrate your attention to the stretches and areas of your body that are not responding to the routines.		Increase reps on push-ups to 20

WEEK 7—A STRETCH TOO FAR?

Some of the progressions are very strong stretches; if you find you are beginning to ache after a stretch session, it maybe that you are not ready for that particular intensity of stretch, so go back to the previous exercises you were comfortable with for a week or two.

7	daily stretch (p15), 20-minute walk, core stability 1, 2, 3, 4, 5, and 6, hamstring stretch, rainbows 5x, glute/piriformis stretch, cobra to upward dog, prone trunk raise, hands at head 5x, push-ups 5x-20, superman on hands and knees 5x, 1 legged bridge 5x, lunge hands up 5x, lunge hands forward and rotate across forward knee 5x, 1 legged squat 5x, standing forward bend to knees, ankles, floor, chest to knees, seated ham stretch, seated glute stretch, seated twist, chest stretch, crucifix 5x, under/over hand clasp, pelvic tilt up to bridge stretch 5x, seated adductor, legs apart, squats 5x, standing quad stretch, standing hamstring stretch, lunge 5x	daily stretch (p15), 20-minute walk, core stability exercise 1 and 3, 45 minutes cardio with 8x 2-minute intervals of brisk pace	daily stretch (p15), 20-minute walk, core stability 1, 2, 3, 4, 5, and 6, hamstring stretch, rainbows 5x, glute/piriformis stretch, cobra to upward dog, prone trunk raise, hands at head 5x, push-ups 5x20, superman on hands and knees 5x, 1 legged bridge 5x, lunge hands up 5x, lunge hands forward and rotate across forward knee 5x, 1 legged squat 5x, standing forward bend to knees, ankles, floor, chest to knees, seated ham stretch, seated glute stretch, seated twist, chest stretch, crucifix 5x, under/over hand clasp, pelvic tilt up to bridge stretch 5x, seated adductor, legs apart, squats 5x, standing quad stretch, standing hamstring stretch, lunge 5x
8	**REPEAT WEEK 7.** Intensify the CV workouts.	introduce 7x 1-minute intervals of hard pace	

THURSDAY	FRIDAY	SATURDAY	SUNDAY
daily stretch (p15), 20-minute walk, core stability exercises 1 and 3, 45 minutes cardio with 8x 2-minute intervals of brisk pace	daily stretch (p15), 20-minute walk, core stability 1, 2, 3, 4, 5, and 6, hamstring stretch, rainbows 5x, glute/piriformis stretch, pelvic tilt 5x, cobra stretch, prone trunk raise 5x, push-ups 10x, seated hamstring stretch, seated glute stretch, seated twist, seated adductor stretch, chest stretch, crucifix 5x, under/over hand clasp, superman 5x, pelvic tilt up to bridge stretch 5x, seated adductor, legs apart, squats 5x, standing quad stretch, standing hamstring stretch, lunge 5x	rest day daily stretch (p15), 20-minute walk	daily stretch(p15), 20-minute walk, core stability exercises 1 and 3, 45 minutes cardio with 8x 2-minute intervals of brisk pace
	Increase reps on push-ups to 20		

TOO MANY REPS?

With strength work increase the number of repetitions so that you are doing two sets of 5–10, then add on more reps so that as you near the end of the second set you have to work harder to complete it. If by the end of the second set you cannot hold the position, you are probably doing too many reps.

daily stretch (p15), 20-minute walk, core stability exercises 1 and 3, 45 minutes cardio with 8x 2-minute intervals of brisk pace	daily stretch (p15), 20-minute walk, core stability 1, 2, 3, 4, 5, and 6, hamstring stretch, rainbows 5x, glute/piriformis stretch, cobra to upward dog, prone trunk raise, hands at head 5x, push-ups 5x 20, superman on hands and knees 5x, 1 legged bridge 5x, lunge hands up 5x, lunge hands forward and rotate across forward knee 5x, 1 legged squat 5x, standing forward bend to knees, ankles, floor, chest to knees, seated hamstring stretch, seated glute stretch, seated twist, chest stretch, crucifix 5x, under/over hand clasp, pelvic tilt up to bridge stretch 5x, seated adductor legs apart, squats 5x, standing quad stretch, standing hamstring stretch, lunge 5x	rest day daily stretch (p15), 20-minute walk	daily stretch (p15), 20-minute walk, core stability exercises 1 and 3, 45 minutes cardio with 8x 2-minute intervals of brisk pace
introduce 7x 1-minute intervals of hard pace			introduce 7x 1-minute intervals of hard pace

5

upper level 1 continued

	MONDAY	TUESDAY	WEDNESDAY
WEEK			
9	daily stretch (p15), 20-minute walk, core stability 1, 2, 3, 4, 5, and 6, hamstring stretch, rainbows 5x, glute/piriformis stretch, cobra to upward dog, prone trunk raise, hands at head 5x, push-ups 5-20x, superman on hands and knees 5x, 1 legged bridge 5x, lunge hands up 5x, lunge hands forward and rotate across forward knee 5x, 1 legged squat 5x, standing forward bend to knees, ankles, floor, chest to knees, seated hamstring stretch, seated glute stretch, seated twist, chest stretch, crucifix 5x, under/over hand clasp, pelvic tilt up to bridge stretch 5x, seated adductor, legs apart, squats 5x, standing quad stretch, standing hamstring stretch, lunge 5x	daily stretch (p15), 20-minute walk, core stability exercises 1 and 3, 50 minutes cardio with 8x-2 minute intervals of brisk pace and 7x 1-minute intervals of hard pace	daily stretch (p15), 20-minute walk, core stability 1, 2, 3, 4, 5, and 6, hamstring stretch, rainbows 5x, glute/piriformis stretch, cobra to upward dog, prone trunk raise, hands at head 5x, push-ups 5-20x, superman on hands and knees 5x, 1 legged bridge 5x, lunge hands up 5x, lunge hands forward and rotate across forward knee 5x, 1 legged squat 5x, standing forward bend to knees, ankles, floor, chest to knees, seated hamstring stretch, seated glute stretch, seated twist, chest stretch, crucifix 5x, under/over hand clasp, pelvic tilt up to bridge stretch 5x, seated adductor, legs apart, squats 5x, standing quad stretch, standing hamstring stretch, lunge 5x
10	**REPEAT WEEK 9** and add camel, prone pigeon, downward dog standing triangles, straight back, forward bend plus rotation, standing balances, tree, if comfortable raise arms, deep squat heels down stretch	**REPEAT WEEK 9**	**REPEAT WEEK 9** and add camel, prone pigeon, downward dog standing triangles, straight back, forward bend plus rotation, standing balances, tree, if comfortable raise arms, deep squat heels down stretch
11 12	daily stretch (p15), 20-minute walk, core stability 1, 2, 3, 4, 5, and 6, hamstring stretch, rainbows 5x, glute/piriformis stretch, cobra to upward dog, prone trunk raise, hands at head 5x, push-ups 5-20x, superman on hands and knees 2x5, 1 legged bridge 2x5, lunge hands up 2x5, lunge hands forward and rotate across forward knee 2x5, 1 legged squat 2x5, standing forward bend to knees, ankles, floor, chest to knees, seated hamstring stretch, seated glute stretch, seated twist, chest stretch, crucifix 5x, under/over hand clasp, pelvic tilt up to bridge stretch 5x, seated adductor, legs apart, squats 5x, standing quad stretch, standing hamstring stretch, lunge 2x5. camel, prone pigeon, downward dog, standing triangles, straight back, forward bend plus rotation, standing balances, tree, deep squat stretch	daily stretch (p15), 20-minute walk, core stability exercises 1 and 3, 50 minutes cardio with 8x-2 minute intervals of brisk pace and 7x 1-minute intervals of hard pace	daily stretch (p15), 20-minute walk, core stability 1, 2, 3, 4, 5, and 6, hamstring stretch, rainbows 5x, glute/piriformis stretch, cobra to upward dog, prone trunk raise, hands at head 5x, push-ups 5-20x, superman on hands and knees 5x, 1 legged bridge 5x, lunge hands up 5x, lunge hands forward and rotate across forward knee 5x, 1 legged squat 5x, standing forward bend to knees, ankles, floor, chest to knees, seated hamstring stretch, seated glute stretch, seated twist, chest stretch, crucifix 5x, under/over hand clasp, pelvic tilt up to bridge stretch 5x, seated adductor, legs apart, squats 5x, standing quad stretch, standing hamstring stretch, lunge 5x, camel, prone pigeon, downward dog, standing triangles, straight back, forward bend plus rotation, standing balances, tree, deep squat stretch

THURSDAY	FRIDAY	SATURDAY	SUNDAY
daily stretch (p15), 20-minute walk, core stability exercises 1 and 3, 50 minutes cardio with 8x 2-minute intervals of brisk pace and 7x 1-minute intervals of hard pace	daily stretch (p15), 20-minute walk, core stability 1, 2, 3, 4, 5, and 6, hamstring stretch, rainbows 5x, glute/piriformis stretch, cobra to upward dog, prone trunk raise, hands at head 5x, push-ups 5-20x, superman on hands and knees 5x, 1 legged bridge 5x, lunge hands up 5x, lunge hands forward and rotate across forward knee 5x, 1 legged squat 5x, standing forward bend to knees, ankles, floor, chest to knees, seated hamstring stretch, seated glute stretch, seated twist, chest stretch, crucifix 5x, under/over hand clasp, pelvic tilt up to bridge stretch 5x, seated adductor, legs apart, squats 5x, standing quad stretch, standing hamstring stretch, lunge 5x	rest day daily stretch (p15), 20-minute walk	daily stretch (p15), 20-minute walk, core stability exercises 1 and 3, 50 minutes cardio with 8x 2-minute intervals of brisk pace and 7x 1-minute intervals of hard pace
REPEAT WEEK 9	**REPEAT WEEK 9** and add camel, prone pigeon, downward dog standing triangles, straight back, forward bend plus rotation, standing balances, tree, if comfortable raise arms, deep squat heels down stretch	**REPEAT WEEK 9**	**REPEAT WEEK 9**
daily stretch (p15), 20-minute walk, core stability exercises 1 and 3, 50 minutes cardio with 8x 2-minute intervals of brisk pace and 7x 1-minute intervals of hard pace	daily stretch (p15), 20-minute walk, core stability 1, 2, 3, 4, 5, and 6, hamstring stretch, rainbows 5x, glute/piriformis stretch, cobra to upward dog, prone trunk raise, hands at head 5x, push-ups 5-20x, superman on hands and knees 5x, 1 legged bridge 5x, lunge hands up 5x, lunge hands forward and rotate across forward knee 5x, 1 legged squat 5x, standing forward bend to knees, ankles, floor, chest to knees, seated hamstring stretch, seated glute stretch, seated twist, chest stretch, crucifix 5x, under/over hand clasp, pelvic tilt up to bridge stretch 5x, seated adductor, legs apart, squats 5x, standing quad stretch, standing hamstring stretch, lunge 5x, camel, prone pigeon, downward dog, standing triangles, straight back, forward bend plus rotation, standing balances, tree, deep squat stretch	rest day daily stretch (p15), 20-minute walk	daily stretch (p15), 20-minute walk, core stability exercises 1 and 3, 50 minutes cardio with 8x 2-minute intervals of brisk pace and 7x 1minute intervals of hard pace

WEEK 11—HOW'S IT GOING?

Increase the repetitions of the strength exercises. If you can comfortably do 2 x 15 repetitions of the body weight lunges and squats, start using some hand weights to add a little more resistance. Don't just focus your attention on the stretches that are easiest for you. The tougher the stretch the more potential it has to balance you.

upper level 2

For people who are in regular intense exercise, maybe five times per week, and want to improve on their flexibility and strength.

WEEK	MONDAY	TUESDAY	WEDNESDAY	
1	daily stretch (p15), 20-minute walk, core stability exercise 1	daily stretch (p15), 20-minute walk, core stability exercise 1	daily stretch (p15), 20-minute walk, core stability exercise 1	
2	daily stretch (p15), 20-minute walk, core stability exercises 1, 2, and 3, supine hamstring stretch, rainbows 5x, glute/piriformis stretch, pelvic tilt 5x, prone cobra, prone trunk raise, arms at side 5x, full push-ups 5-10x, seated hamstrings stretch, seated glute stretch, seated twist, seated adductor stretch, standing straight arms forward back up push away, crucifix 5x, under/over hand clasp	daily stretch (p15), 20-minute walk, core stability exercise 1, 50 minutes cardio with 8x 2-minute intervals of brisk pace	daily stretch (p15), 20-minute walk, core stability exercises 1, 2, and 3, supine hamstring stretch, rainbows 5x, glute/piriformis stretch, pelvic tilt 5x, prone cobra, prone trunk raise, arms at side 5x, full push-ups 5-10x, seated hamstrings stretch, seated glute stretch, seated twist, seated adductor stretch, standing straight arms forward back up push away, crucifix 5x, under/over hand clasp	
3	**REPEAT WEEK 2** and add prone superman 5x, pelvic tilt and curl up to bridge 5x, seated adductor legs apart, squats, heels down, knees to 90 5x, standing quadriceps stretch, standing hamstrings stretch, lunge hands on knee or hips 5x, core exercises 4 and 5	**REPEAT WEEK 2** and add core stability exercise 3	**REPEAT WEEK 2** and add prone superman 5x, pelvic tilt and curl up to bridge 5x, seated adductor legs apart, squats, heels down, knees to 90 5x, standing quadriceps stretch, standing hamstrings stretch, lunge hands on knee or hips 5x, core exercises 4 and 5	
4	daily stretch (p15), 20-minute walk, core stability exercises 1 2, 3, 4, 5, and 6, supine hamstring stretch, rainbows 5x, glute/piriformis stretch, cobra, prone trunk raise 2x5, full push-ups 2x5-10, seated hamstrings stretch, sitting glute stretch, seated twist, seated adductor, chest stretch, crucifix 5x, under/over hand clasp, superman 2x5, pelvic tilt and curl up to bridge 2x5, sitting adductor legs apart, squats, heels down, knees to 90 2x5, standing quadriceps stretch, standing hamstrings stretch, lunge hands on knee or hips 2x5	daily stretch (p15), 20-minute walk, core stability exercises 1, and 3, 50 minutes cardio with 8x 2-minute intervals of brisk pace	daily stretch (p15), 20-minute walk, core stability exercises 1 2, 3, 4, 5, and 6, supine hamstring stretch, rainbows 5x, glute/piriformis stretch, cobra, prone trunk raise 2x5, full push-ups 2x5-10, seated hamstrings stretch, sitting glute stretch, seated twist, seated adductor, chest stretch, crucifix 5x, under/over hand clasp, superman 2x5, pelvic tilt and curl up to bridge 2x5, sitting adductor legs apart, squats, heels down, knees to 90 2x5, standing quadriceps stretch, standing hamstrings stretch, lunge hands on knee or hips 2x5	

THE RIGHT STRETCH

If your current program features some sports-specific stretches, you may want to try adding them to the daily stretches. The aim of this schedule is to increase suppleness and build up strength to help reduce the risk of injuries during your training sessions.

THURSDAY	FRIDAY	SATURDAY	SUNDAY
daily stretch (p15), 20-minute walk, core stability exercise 1	daily stretch (p15), 20-minute walk, core stability exercise 1	rest day daily stretch (p15), 20-minute walk	daily stretch (p15), 20-minute walk, core stability exercise 1
daily stretch (p15), 20-minute walk, core stability exercise 1, 50 minutes cardio with 8x 2-minute intervals of brisk pace	daily stretch (p15), 20-minute walk, core stability exercises 1, 2, and 3, supine hamstring stretch, rainbows 5x, glute/piriformis stretch, pelvic tilt 5x, prone cobra, prone trunk raise, arms at side 5x, full push-ups 5-10x, seated hamstrings stretch, seated glute stretch, seated twist, seated adductor stretch, standing straight arms forward back up push away, crucifix 5x, under/over hand clasp	rest day daily stretch(p15), 20-minute walk	daily stretch (p15), 20-minute walk, core stability exercise 1, 50 minutes cardio with 8x 2-minute intervals of brisk pace
REPEAT WEEK 2 and add core stability exercise 3	**REPEAT WEEK 2** and add prone superman 5x, pelvic tilt and curl up to bridge 5x, seated adductor legs apart, squats, heels down, knees to 90 5x, standing quadriceps stretch, standing hamstrings stretch, lunge hands on knee or hips 5x, core exercises 4 and 5	**REPEAT WEEK 2**	**REPEAT WEEK 2** and add core stability exercise 3
daily stretch (p15), 20-minute walk, core stability exercises 1 and 3, 50 minutes cardio with 8x 2-minute intervals of brisk pace	daily stretch (p15), 20-minute walk, core stability exercises 1 2, 3, 4, 5, and 6, supine hamstring stretch, rainbows 5x, glute/piriformis stretch, cobra, prone trunk raise, 2x5, full push-ups 2x5-10, seated hamstrings stretch, seated glute stretch, seated twist, seated adductor, chest stretch, crucifix 5x, under/over hand clasp, superman 2x5, pelvic tilt and curl up to bridge 2x5 sitting adductor legs apart, squats, heels down, knees to 90 2x5, standing quadriceps stretch, standing hamstrings stretch, lunge hands on knee or hips 2x5	rest day daily stretch (p15), 20-minute walk	daily stretch (p15), 20-minute walk, core stability exercises 1 and 3, 50 minutes cardio with 8x 2-minute intervals of brisk pace

6

upper level 2 continued

WEEK	MONDAY	TUESDAY	WEDNESDAY
5	daily stretch (p15), 20-minute walk, core stability exercises 1, 2, 3, 4, and 5, supine hamstring stretch, rainbows 5x, glute/piriformis stretch, prone cobra, seated hamstrings stretch, seated glute stretch, seated twist, seated adductor, chest stretch, crucifix 5x, under/over hand clasp, seated adductor, squats 2x5, standing quadriceps stretch, standing hamstrings stretch, cobra to upward dog, prone trunk raise 5x, push-ups 2x5-10, superman on hands and knees 5x, 1 legged bridge 5x, lunge hands up 5x, lunge hands forward and rotate across forward knee 5x, 1 legged squat 5x, standing forward bend	daily stretch (p15), 20-minute walk, core stability exercises 1 and 3, 50 minutes cardio with 8x 2-minute intervals of brisk pace	daily stretch (p15), 20-minute walk, core stability exercises 1, 2, 3, 4, and 5, supine hamstring stretch, rainbows 5x, glute/piriformis stretch, prone cobra, seated hamstrings stretch, seated glute stretch, seated twist, seated adductor, chest stretch, crucifix 5x, under/over hand clasp, seated adductor, squats 2x5, standing quadriceps stretch, standing hamstrings stretch, cobra to upward dog, prone trunk raise 5x, push-ups 2x5-10, superman on hands and knees 5x, 1 legged bridge 5x, lunge hands up 5x, lunge hands forward and rotate across forward knee 5x, 1 legged squat 5x, standing forward bend
6	**ENDURANCE WEEK REPEAT WEEK 5**	**REPEAT WEEK 5** increase cardio to 75 minutes with 3 x 5-min intervals	**REPEAT WEEK 5**
7	daily stretch (p15), 20-minute walk, core stability exercises 1, 2, 3, 4, and 5, supine hamstring stretch, rainbows 5x, glute/piriformis stretch, prone cobra, camel, prone pigeon, seated hamstrings stretch, seated glute stretch, seated twist, seated adductor, chest stretch, crucifix 5x, under/over hand clasp, seated adductor, squats 2x5, standing quadriceps stretch, standing hamstrings stretch, cobra to upward dog, downward dog, prone trunk raise 5x, push-ups 2x5-10, superman on hands and knees 5x, 1 legged bridge 5x, lunge hands up 5x, lunge hands forward and rotate across forward knee 5x, 1 legged squat 5x, standing forward bend, tree, deep squat stretch	daily stretch (p15), 20-minute walk, core stability exercises 1 and 3, 75 minutes cardio at endurance pace with 3x 5-minute intervals of brisk pace	daily stretch (p15), 20-minute walk, core stability exercises 1, 2, 3, 4, and 5, supine hamstring stretch, rainbows 5x, glute/piriformis stretch, prone cobra, camel, prone pigeon, seated hamstrings stretch, seated glute stretch, seated twist, seated adductor, chest stretch, crucifix 5x, under/over hand clasp, seated adductor, squats 2x5, standing quadriceps stretch, standing hamstrings stretch, cobra to upward dog, downward dog, prone trunk raise 5x, push-ups 2x5-10, superman on hands and knees 5x, 1 legged bridge 5x, lunge hands up 5x, lunge hands forward and rotate across forward knee 5x, 1 legged squat 5x, standing forward bend, tree, deep squat stretch

8

REPEAT WEEK 7
Progress the duration and depth of your stretches; focus on particular areas that seem less responsive. You may wish to try some of the more difficult stretches on a less intense but daily basis. Where comfortable increase the repetitions of strength work.

THURSDAY	FRIDAY	SATURDAY	SUNDAY
daily stretch (p15), 20-minute walk, core stability exercises 1 and 3, 50 minutes cardio with 8x 2-minute intervals of brisk pace	daily stretch (p15), 20-minute walk, core stability exercises 1, 2, 3, 4, and 5, supine hamstring stretch, rainbows 5x, glute/piriformis stretch, prone cobra, seated hamstrings stretch, seated glute stretch, seated twist, seated adductor, chest stretch, crucifix 5x, under/over hand clasp, seated adductor, squats 2x5, standing quadriceps stretch, standing hamstrings stretch, cobra to upward dog, prone trunk raise 5x, push-ups 2x5-10, superman on hands and knees 5x, 1 legged bridge 5x, lunge hands up 5x, lunge hands forward and rotate across forward knee 5x, 1 legged squat 5x, standing forward bend	rest day daily stretch (p15), 20-minute walk	daily stretch (p15), 20-minute walk, core stability exercises 1 and 3, 50 minutes cardio with 8x 2-minute intervals of brisk pace
REPEAT WEEK 5 increase cardio to 60 minutes with 3 x 5-min intervals	**REPEAT WEEK 5**	**REPEAT WEEK 5**	**REPEAT WEEK 5** increase cardio to 90 minutes with 3x 5-min intervals
daily stretch (p15), 20-minute walk, core stability exercises 1 and 3, 60 minutes cardio at endurance pace with 3x 5-minute intervals of brisk pace	daily stretch (p15), 20-minute walk, core stability exercises 1, 2, 3, 4, and 5, supine hamstring stretch, rainbows 5x, glute/piriformis stretch, prone cobra, camel, prone pigeon, seated hamstrings stretch, seated glute stretch, seated twist, seated adductor, chest stretch, crucifix 5x, under/over hand clasp, seated adductor, squats 2x5, standing quadriceps stretch, standing hamstrings stretch, cobra to upward dog, downward dog, prone trunk raise 5x, push-ups 2x5-10, superman on hands and knees 5x, 1 legged bridge 5x, lunge hands up 5x, lunge hands forward and rotate across forward knee 5x, 1 legged squat 5x, standing forward bend, tree, deep squat stretch	rest day daily stretch (p15), 20-minute walk	daily stretch (p15), 20-minute walk, core stability exercises 1 and 3, 90 minutes cardio with 3x 5-minute intervals of brisk pace
REPEAT WEEK 7	**REPEAT WEEK 7**	**REPEAT WEEK 7**	**REPEAT WEEK 7**

6

upper level 2 continued

WEEK	MONDAY	TUESDAY	WEDNESDAY	
9	daily stretch (p15), 20-minute walk, core stability exercises 1, 2, 3, 4, and 5, supine hamstring stretch, rainbows 5x, glute/piriformis stretch, prone cobra, camel, prone pigeon, seated hamstrings stretch, seated glute stretch, seated twist, seated adductor, chest stretch, crucifix 5x, under/over hand clasp, seated adductor, squats 2x10, standing quadriceps stretch, standing hamstrings stretch, cobra to upward dog, downward dog, prone trunk raise 2x5, push-ups 2x10-20, superman on hands and knees 2x5, 1 legged bridge 2x5, lunge hands up 2x5, lunge hands forward and rotate across forward knee 5x, 1 legged squat 2x5, standing forward bend, tree, deep squat stretch	daily stretch (p15), 20-minute walk, core stability exercises 1 and 3, 60 minutes cardio with 8x 2-minute intervals of brisk pace	daily stretch (p15), 20-minute walk, core stability exercises 1, 2, 3, 4, and 5, supine hamstring stretch, rainbows 5x, glute/piriformis stretch, prone cobra, camel, prone pigeon, seated hamstrings stretch, seated glute stretch, seated twist, seated adductor, chest stretch, crucifix 5x, under/over hand clasp, seated adductor, squats 2x10, standing quadriceps stretch, standing hamstrings stretch, cobra to upward dog, downward dog, prone trunk raise 2x5, push-ups 2x10-20, superman on hands and knees 2x5, 1 legged bridge 2x5, lunge hands up 2x5, lunge hands forward and rotate across forward knee 5x, 1 legged squat 2x5, standing forward bend, tree, deep squat stretch	
10	**CONSOLIDATION WEEK** **REPEAT WEEK 9**	**REPEAT WEEK 9**	**REPEAT WEEK 9**	
11	daily stretch (p15), 20-minute walk, core stability exercises 1, 2, 3, 4, and 5, supine hamstring stretch, rainbows 5x, glute/piriformis stretch, prone cobra, camel, prone pigeon, seated hamstrings stretch, seated glute stretch, seated twist, seated adductor, chest stretch, crucifix 5x, under/over hand clasp, seated adductor, squats 2x15, standing quadriceps stretch, standing hamstrings stretch, cobra to upward dog, downward dog, prone trunk raise 3x5, push-ups 3x10-20, superman on hands and knees 3x5, 1 legged bridge 3x5, lunge hands up 2x10, lunge hands forward and rotate across forward knee 2x10, 1 legged squat 2x10, standing forward bend, tree, deep squat stretch	daily stretch (p15), 20-minute walk, core stability exercises 1 and 3, 75 minutes cardio at endurance pace with 5x 4-minute intervals of steady pace	daily stretch (p15), 20-minute walk, core stability exercises 1, 2, 3, 4, and 5, supine hamstring stretch, rainbows 5x, glute/piriformis stretch, prone cobra, camel, prone pigeon, seated hamstrings stretch, seated glute stretch, seated twist, seated adductor, chest stretch, crucifix 5x, under/over hand clasp, seated adductor, squats 2x15, standing quadriceps stretch, standing hamstrings stretch, cobra to upward dog, downward dog, prone trunk raise 3x5, push-ups 3x10-20, superman on hands and knees 3x5, 1 legged bridge 3x5, lunge hands up 2x10, lunge hands forward and rotate across forward knee 2x10, 1 legged squat 2x10, standing forward bend, tree, deep squat stretch	
12	**REPEAT WEEK 11** Add standing warrior poses with side bends, forward bends and hip rotation, and walking lunges		**REPEAT WEEK 11**	

THURSDAY	FRIDAY	SATURDAY	SUNDAY
daily stretch (p15), 20-minute walk, core stability exercises 1 and 3, 60 minutes cardio with 8x 2-minute intervals of brisk pace	daily stretch (p15), 20-minute walk, core stability exercises 1, 2, 3, 4, and 5, supine hamstring stretch, rainbows 5x, glute/piriformis stretch, prone cobra, camel, prone pigeon, seated hamstrings stretch, seated glute stretch, seated twist, seated adductor, chest stretch, crucifix 5x, under/over hand clasp, seated adductor, squats 2x10, standing quadriceps stretch, standing hamstrings stretch, cobra to upward dog, downward dog, prone trunk raise 2x5, push-ups 2x10-20, superman on hands and knees 2x5, 1 legged bridge 2x5, lunge hands up 2x5, lunge hands forward and rotate across forward knee 5x, 1 legged squat 2x5, standing forward bend, tree, deep squat stretch	rest day daily stretch (p15), 20-minute walk	daily stretch (p15), 20-minute walk, core stability exercises 1 and 3, 90 minutes cardio at endurance pace
REPEAT WEEK 9	**REPEAT WEEK 9**	**REPEAT WEEK 9**	**REPEAT WEEK 9**
daily stretch (p15), 20-minute walk, core stability exercises 1 and 3, 50 minutes cardio at steady pace with 8x 2-minute intervals of brisk pace and 7x1-hard pace	daily stretch (p15), 20-minute walk, core stability exercises 1, 2, 3, 4, and 5, supine hamstring stretch, rainbows 5x, glute/piriformis stretch, prone cobra, camel, prone pigeon, seated hamstrings stretch, seated glute stretch, seated twist, seated adductor, chest stretch, crucifix 5x, under/over hand clasp, seated adductor, squats 2x15, standing quadriceps stretch, standing hamstrings stretch, cobra to upward dog, downward dog, prone trunk raise 3x5, push-ups 3x10-20, superman on hands and knees 3x5, 1 legged bridge 3x5, lunge hands up 2x10, lunge hands forward and rotate across forward knee 2x10, 1 legged squat 2x10, standing forward bend, tree, deep squat stretch	rest day daily stretch (p15), 20-minute walk	daily stretch (p15), 20-minute walk, core stability exercises 1 and 3, 105 minutes cardio at endurance pace
REPEAT WEEK 11	**REPEAT WEEK 11**	**REPEAT WEEK 11**	**REPEAT WEEK 11**

6

upper level 2 continued

WEEK	MONDAY	TUESDAY	WEDNESDAY	
13	daily stretch (p15), 20-minute walk, core stability exercises 1, 2, 3, 4, and 5, supine hamstring stretch, rainbows 5x, glute/piriformis, prone cobra, seated hamstrings stretch, seated glute stretch, seated twist, seated adductor stretch, chest stretch, crucifix 5x, under/over hand clasp, seated adductor legs apart, squats 10x, standing quadriceps stretch, standing hamstrings stretch, cobra to upward dog, prone trunk raise 3x5, push-ups 2x10, superman on hands and knees 3x5, 1 legged bridge 3x5, lunge hands up 2x5, lunge hands forward and rotate across forward knee2x5, 1 legged squat 2x5, standing forward bend, camel , prone pigeon , downward dog, standing triangles, straight back, forward bend plus rotation, tree, deep squat stretch, standing warrior poses with side bends, forward bends, and hip rotation, walking lunges	daily stretch (p15), 20-minute walk, core stability exercises 1 and 3, 75 minutes cardio at endurance pace with 5x 4-minute intervals of steady pace	daily stretch (p15), 20-minute walk, core stability exercises 1, 2, 3, 4, and 5, supine hamstring stretch, rainbows 5x, glute/piriformis, prone cobra, seated hamstrings stretch, seated glute stretch, seated twist, seated adductor stretch, chest stretch, crucifix 5x, under/over hand clasp, seated adductor legs apart, squats 2x15, standing quadriceps stretch, standing hamstrings stretch, cobra to upward dog, prone trunk raise 3x5, push-ups 3x15, superman on hands and knees 3x5, 1 legged bridge 3x5, lunge hands up 2x10, lunge hands forward and rotate across forward knee2x10, one-legged squat 2x10, standing forward bend, camel , prone pigeon , downward dog, standing triangles, straight back, forward bend plus rotation, tree, deep squat stretch, standing warrior poses with side bends, forward bends, and hip rotation, walking lunges	
14	REPEAT WEEK 13	REPEAT WEEK 13 reduce cardio to 60 minutes	REPEAT WEEK 13	
15	REPEAT WEEK 14	REPEAT WEEK 14 increase cardio to 75 minutes	REPEAT WEEK 14	
16	REPEAT WEEK 15 Try to keep variety going in your cardio workouts; doing the same thing repeatedly can take the pleasure out of it. Find a training buddy; this can give you that added incentive to manitain your training schedules.		REPEAT WEEK 15	

ADD JUMP POWER TO YOUR ROUTINE

Plyometrics or jumping is a great way to increase explosive power. Add these exercises to your routines for Monday, Wednesday, and Friday. Jump up and down onto a SOLID STEADY platform no more than one-half knee height. Jumping forward and backward 8x, hopping forward 8x, push-ups with clapping 8x.

THURSDAY	FRIDAY	SATURDAY	SUNDAY
daily stretch (p15), 20-minute walk, core stability exercises 1, and 3, 50 minutes cardio at steady pace with 8x 2-minute intervals of brisk and 7x 1-minute hard pace	daily stretch (p15), 20-minute walk, core stability exercises 1, 2, 3, 4, and 5, supine hamstring stretch, rainbows 5x, glute/piriformis, prone cobra, seated hamstrings stretch, seated glute stretch, seated twist, seated adductor stretch, chest stretch, crucifix 5x, under/over hand clasp, seated adductor legs apart, squats 10x, standing quadriceps stretch, standing hamstrings stretch, cobra to upward dog, prone trunk raise 3x5, push-ups 2x10, superman on hands and knees 3x5, 1 legged bridge 3x5, lunge hands up 2x5, lunge hands forward and rotate across forward knee2x5, 1 legged squat 2x5, standing forward bend, camel , prone pigeon , downward dog, standing triangles, straight back, forward bend plus rotation, tree, deep squat stretch, standing warrior poses with side bends, forward bends, and hip rotation, walking lunges	rest day daily stretch (p15), 20-minute walk	daily stretch (p15), 20-minute walk, core stability exercises 1 and 3, 105 minutes cardio at endurance pace
REPEAT WEEK 13 reduce cardio to 50 minutes	**REPEAT WEEK 13**	**REPEAT WEEK 13**	**REPEAT WEEK 13** reduce cardio to 90 minutes
REPEAT WEEK 14 increase cardio to 60 minutes	**REPEAT WEEK 14**	**REPEAT WEEK 14**	**REPEAT WEEK 14** increase cardio to 105 minutes
REPEAT WEEK 15 reduce cardio to 50 minutes	**REPEAT WEEK 14**	**REPEAT WEEK 15**	**REPEAT WEEK 15** reduce cardio to 90 minutes

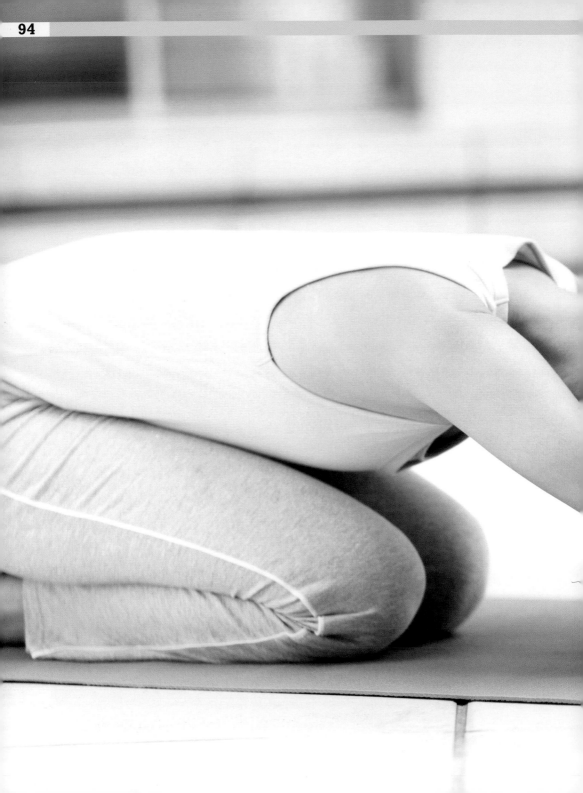

stretching diary

Keeping a record of your stretching routines and cardio exercises can be instrumental in helping you discover how to improve your fitness. You will be able to see at a glance when you felt your best, what the conditions were, and what you ate and drank before and during your exercise sessions, and you will be able to monitor your progress through the schedules as you get fitter, stronger, and more flexible.

WEEK 1

DATE

OBJECTIVES

MONDAY

STRETCHES

1
2
3
4
5
6
7
8
9
10
11

STRETCH COMMENTS

CARDIO

TIME/DISTANCE	COMMENTS

HOW DO YOU FEEL

BEFORE THE SESSION

AFTER THE SESSION

TUESDAY

STRETCHES

1
2
3
4
5
6
7
8
9
10
11

STRETCH COMMENTS

CARDIO

TIME/DISTANCE	COMMENTS

HOW DO YOU FEEL

BEFORE THE SESSION

AFTER THE SESSION

WEDNESDAY

STRETCHES

1	
2	
3	
4	
5	
6	
7	
8	
9	
10	
11	

STRETCH COMMENTS

CARDIO

TIME/DISTANCE	COMMENTS

HOW DO YOU FEEL

BEFORE THE SESSION

AFTER THE SESSION

THURSDAY

STRETCHES

1	
2	
3	
4	
5	
6	
7	
8	
9	
10	
11	

STRETCH COMMENTS

CARDIO

TIME/DISTANCE	COMMENTS

HOW DO YOU FEEL

BEFORE THE SESSION

AFTER THE SESSION

diet notes

Never force a stretch beyond the point of mild tension. Stretching is not meant to be painful; it should be relaxing and very beneficial. It is a mistake to think that you have to feel pain to get the most out of your stretching.

Time to stretch?

Stretching exercises are performed best when the body and muscles have had sufficient time to warm up and loosen. Allow at least an hour after getting out of bed before engaging in any type of exercise.

diet notes

FRIDAY

STRETCHES	
1	
2	
3	
4	
5	
6	
7	
8	
9	
10	
11	

STRETCH COMMENTS

CARDIO

TIME/DISTANCE	COMMENTS

HOW DO YOU FEEL

BEFORE THE SESSION

AFTER THE SESSION

SATURDAY

STRETCHES	
1	
2	
3	
4	
5	
6	
7	
8	
9	
10	
11	

STRETCH COMMENTS

CARDIO

TIME/DISTANCE	COMMENTS

HOW DO YOU FEEL

BEFORE THE SESSION

AFTER THE SESSION

SUNDAY

STRETCHES	
1	
2	
3	
4	
5	
6	
7	
8	
9	
10	
11	

STRETCH COMMENTS

CARDIO

TIME/DISTANCE	COMMENTS

HOW DO YOU FEEL

BEFORE THE SESSION

AFTER THE SESSION

comments

WEEKLY SUMMARY   DATE

GOALS MET

GOALS EXCEEDED

NEXT WEEK

STRETCHING NOTES

CARDIO NOTES

DIETARY NOTES

WEEK 2

DATE

OBJECTIVES

_____
_____
_____

MONDAY

STRETCHES	
1	
2	
3	
4	
5	
6	
7	
8	
9	
10	
11	

STRETCH COMMENTS

CARDIO

TIME/DISTANCE	COMMENTS

HOW DO YOU FEEL

BEFORE THE SESSION

AFTER THE SESSION

TUESDAY

STRETCHES	
1	
2	
3	
4	
5	
6	
7	
8	
9	
10	
11	

STRETCH COMMENTS

CARDIO

TIME/DISTANCE	COMMENTS

HOW DO YOU FEEL

BEFORE THE SESSION

AFTER THE SESSION

WEDNESDAY

STRETCHES

1	
2	
3	
4	
5	
6	
7	
8	
9	
10	
11	

STRETCH COMMENTS

CARDIO

TIME/DISTANCE	COMMENTS

HOW DO YOU FEEL

BEFORE THE SESSION

AFTER THE SESSION

THURSDAY

STRETCHES

1	
2	
3	
4	
5	
6	
7	
8	
9	
10	
11	

STRETCH COMMENTS

CARDIO

TIME/DISTANCE	COMMENTS

HOW DO YOU FEEL

BEFORE THE SESSION

AFTER THE SESSION

diet notes

Be consistent with your stretching routine. Stretch regularly each day and you will gradually build flexibility and range of motion. You will not feel the benefits of your routine if you stretch only once a week.

Keep flexing

The flexibility of your body changes from day to day, so don't be concerned if you are not able to perform the stretching routines to exactly the same standard at each session. You will notice the difference once you complete a level.

diet notes

FRIDAY

STRETCHES	
1	
2	
3	
4	
5	
6	
7	
8	
9	
10	
11	

STRETCH COMMENTS

CARDIO

TIME/DISTANCE	COMMENTS

HOW DO YOU FEEL
BEFORE THE SESSION

AFTER THE SESSION

SATURDAY

STRETCHES	
1	
2	
3	
4	
5	
6	
7	
8	
9	
10	
11	

STRETCH COMMENTS

CARDIO

TIME/DISTANCE	COMMENTS

HOW DO YOU FEEL
BEFORE THE SESSION

AFTER THE SESSION

SUNDAY

STRETCHES

1	
2	
3	
4	
5	
6	
7	
8	
9	
10	
11	

STRETCH COMMENTS

CARDIO

TIME/DISTANCE	COMMENTS

HOW DO YOU FEEL

BEFORE THE SESSION

AFTER THE SESSION

comments

WEEKLY SUMMARY DATE

GOALS MET

GOALS EXCEEDED

NEXT WEEK

STRETCHING NOTES

CARDIO NOTES

DIETARY NOTES

WEEK 3

DATE

OBJECTIVES

_____
_____
_____

MONDAY

STRETCHES

1	
2	
3	
4	
5	
6	
7	
8	
9	
10	
11	

STRETCH COMMENTS

CARDIO

TIME/DISTANCE	COMMENTS

HOW DO YOU FEEL

BEFORE THE SESSION

AFTER THE SESSION

TUESDAY

STRETCHES

1	
2	
3	
4	
5	
6	
7	
8	
9	
10	
11	

STRETCH COMMENTS

CARDIO

TIME/DISTANCE	COMMENTS

HOW DO YOU FEEL

BEFORE THE SESSION

AFTER THE SESSION

WEDNESDAY

STRETCHES

1	
2	
3	
4	
5	
6	
7	
8	
9	
10	
11	

STRETCH COMMENTS

CARDIO

TIME/DISTANCE	COMMENTS

HOW DO YOU FEEL

BEFORE THE SESSION

AFTER THE SESSION

THURSDAY

STRETCHES

1	
2	
3	
4	
5	
6	
7	
8	
9	
10	
11	

STRETCH COMMENTS

CARDIO

TIME/DISTANCE	COMMENTS

HOW DO YOU FEEL

BEFORE THE SESSION

AFTER THE SESSION

diet notes

Regular stretching activates fluids in your joints, thereby reducing the wear and tear caused by friction. Increased water intake is also believed to contribute to increased mobility for tissues and joints that have become less supple.

Relax into the stretch

Flexibility provides anti-aging benefits that may keep you feeling fit and young. Remember to cool down after each session. Stretching should be peaceful, both physically and mentally. Quiet your mind, breathe deeply, and let yourself relax.

diet notes

FRIDAY

STRETCHES	
1	
2	
3	
4	
5	
6	
7	
8	
9	
10	
11	

STRETCH COMMENTS

CARDIO

TIME/DISTANCE	COMMENTS

HOW DO YOU FEEL
BEFORE THE SESSION

AFTER THE SESSION

SATURDAY

STRETCHES	
1	
2	
3	
4	
5	
6	
7	
8	
9	
10	
11	

STRETCH COMMENTS

CARDIO

TIME/DISTANCE	COMMENTS

HOW DO YOU FEEL
BEFORE THE SESSION

AFTER THE SESSION

SUNDAY

STRETCHES	
1	
2	
3	
4	
5	
6	
7	
8	
9	
10	
11	

STRETCH COMMENTS

CARDIO

TIME/DISTANCE	COMMENTS

HOW DO YOU FEEL

BEFORE THE SESSION

AFTER THE SESSION

comments

WEEKLY SUMMARY DATE

GOALS MET

GOALS EXCEEDED

NEXT WEEK

STRETCHING NOTES

CARDIO NOTES

DIETARY NOTES

WEEK 4

DATE

OBJECTIVES
_____
_____
_____

MONDAY

STRETCHES

1	
2	
3	
4	
5	
6	
7	
8	
9	
10	
11	

STRETCH COMMENTS

CARDIO

TIME/DISTANCE	COMMENTS

HOW DO YOU FEEL
BEFORE THE SESSION

AFTER THE SESSION

TUESDAY

STRETCHES

1	
2	
3	
4	
5	
6	
7	
8	
9	
10	
11	

STRETCH COMMENTS

CARDIO

TIME/DISTANCE	COMMENTS

HOW DO YOU FEEL
BEFORE THE SESSION

AFTER THE SESSION

WEDNESDAY

STRETCHES

1	
2	
3	
4	
5	
6	
7	
8	
9	
10	
11	

STRETCH COMMENTS

CARDIO

TIME/DISTANCE	COMMENTS

HOW DO YOU FEEL

BEFORE THE SESSION

AFTER THE SESSION

THURSDAY

STRETCHES

1	
2	
3	
4	
5	
6	
7	
8	
9	
10	
11	

STRETCH COMMENTS

CARDIO

TIME/DISTANCE	COMMENTS

HOW DO YOU FEEL

BEFORE THE SESSION

AFTER THE SESSION

diet notes

Set training goals. Training goals eventually lead to competition success. Pro athletes leave reminders of these goals in clearly visible places. Every morning they are reminded of where they want to be.

Keep it different

Repeating the same kind of routine day in, day out, can take the pleasure out of your exercise. Try taking different routes when doing your cardio exercise and mix and match your stretches to keep it fresh.

diet notes

FRIDAY

STRETCHES	
1	
2	
3	
4	
5	
6	
7	
8	
9	
10	
11	

STRETCH COMMENTS

CARDIO

TIME/DISTANCE	COMMENTS

HOW DO YOU FEEL
BEFORE THE SESSION

AFTER THE SESSION

SATURDAY

STRETCHES	
1	
2	
3	
4	
5	
6	
7	
8	
9	
10	
11	

STRETCH COMMENTS

CARDIO

TIME/DISTANCE	COMMENTS

HOW DO YOU FEEL
BEFORE THE SESSION

AFTER THE SESSION

SUNDAY

STRETCHES

1	
2	
3	
4	
5	
6	
7	
8	
9	
10	
11	

STRETCH COMMENTS

CARDIO

TIME/DISTANCE	COMMENTS

HOW DO YOU FEEL
BEFORE THE SESSION

AFTER THE SESSION

comments

WEEKLY SUMMARY   DATE

GOALS MET	
GOALS EXCEEDED	
NEXT WEEK	

STRETCHING NOTES

CARDIO NOTES

DIETARY NOTES

WEEK 5

DATE

OBJECTIVES

_____
_____
_____

MONDAY

STRETCHES

1	
2	
3	
4	
5	
6	
7	
8	
9	
10	
11	

STRETCH COMMENTS

CARDIO

TIME/DISTANCE	COMMENTS

HOW DO YOU FEEL

BEFORE THE SESSION

AFTER THE SESSION

TUESDAY

STRETCHES

1	
2	
3	
4	
5	
6	
7	
8	
9	
10	
11	

STRETCH COMMENTS

CARDIO

TIME/DISTANCE	COMMENTS

HOW DO YOU FEEL

BEFORE THE SESSION

AFTER THE SESSION

WEDNESDAY

STRETCHES

1	
2	
3	
4	
5	
6	
7	
8	
9	
10	
11	

STRETCH COMMENTS

CARDIO

TIME/DISTANCE	COMMENTS

HOW DO YOU FEEL

BEFORE THE SESSION

AFTER THE SESSION

THURSDAY

STRETCHES

1	
2	
3	
4	
5	
6	
7	
8	
9	
10	
11	

STRETCH COMMENTS

CARDIO

TIME/DISTANCE	COMMENTS

HOW DO YOU FEEL

BEFORE THE SESSION

AFTER THE SESSION

diet notes

Training gear for cold winter nights can be hard to choose. You want to be warm but not sweat excessively. Choose a lightweight running jacket (get a showerproof, windproof one), tights, and a thermal top, made from "wicking" material.

boost your energy

Try to eat within an hour of finishing your workout. The best way to reenergize is to drink plenty of fluids and to eat a meal high in carbohydrates and a 30-percent protein content.

diet notes

FRIDAY

STRETCHES

1	
2	
3	
4	
5	
6	
7	
8	
9	
10	
11	

STRETCH COMMENTS

CARDIO

TIME/DISTANCE	COMMENTS

HOW DO YOU FEEL

BEFORE THE SESSION

AFTER THE SESSION

SATURDAY

STRETCHES

1	
2	
3	
4	
5	
6	
7	
8	
9	
10	
11	

STRETCH COMMENTS

CARDIO

TIME/DISTANCE	COMMENTS

HOW DO YOU FEEL

BEFORE THE SESSION

AFTER THE SESSION

SUNDAY

STRETCHES

1	
2	
3	
4	
5	
6	
7	
8	
9	
10	
11	

STRETCH COMMENTS

CARDIO

TIME/DISTANCE	COMMENTS

HOW DO YOU FEEL

BEFORE THE SESSION

AFTER THE SESSION

comments

WEEKLY SUMMARY   DATE

GOALS MET

GOALS EXCEEDED

NEXT WEEK

STRETCHING NOTES

CARDIO NOTES

DIETARY NOTES

WEEK 6

DATE

OBJECTIVES

_____
_____
_____

MONDAY

STRETCHES

1	
2	
3	
4	
5	
6	
7	
8	
9	
10	
11	

STRETCH COMMENTS

CARDIO

TIME/DISTANCE	COMMENTS

HOW DO YOU FEEL

BEFORE THE SESSION

AFTER THE SESSION

TUESDAY

STRETCHES

1	
2	
3	
4	
5	
6	
7	
8	
9	
10	
11	

STRETCH COMMENTS

CARDIO

TIME/DISTANCE	COMMENTS

HOW DO YOU FEEL

BEFORE THE SESSION

AFTER THE SESSION

WEDNESDAY

STRETCHES

1	
2	
3	
4	
5	
6	
7	
8	
9	
10	
11	

STRETCH COMMENTS

CARDIO

TIME/DISTANCE	COMMENTS

HOW DO YOU FEEL

BEFORE THE SESSION

AFTER THE SESSION

THURSDAY

STRETCHES

1	
2	
3	
4	
5	
6	
7	
8	
9	
10	
11	

STRETCH COMMENTS

CARDIO

TIME/DISTANCE	COMMENTS

HOW DO YOU FEEL

BEFORE THE SESSION

AFTER THE SESSION

diet notes

Getting from where you are now to where you want to be requires you to have a specific drive. You need enthusiasm, a dream, and a goal, and you also need to recognize that you have to be willing to work for your success.

all change

Your body quickly adapts to routine, which can minimize the effectiveness of your workouts. To keep your training fresh, try different training ideas, such as increasing the reps and reducing the sets.

diet notes

FRIDAY

STRETCHES	
1	
2	
3	
4	
5	
6	
7	
8	
9	
10	
11	

STRETCH COMMENTS

CARDIO

TIME/DISTANCE	COMMENTS

HOW DO YOU FEEL
BEFORE THE SESSION

AFTER THE SESSION

SATURDAY

STRETCHES	
1	
2	
3	
4	
5	
6	
7	
8	
9	
10	
11	

STRETCH COMMENTS

CARDIO

TIME/DISTANCE	COMMENTS

HOW DO YOU FEEL
BEFORE THE SESSION

AFTER THE SESSION

SUNDAY

STRETCHES

1	
2	
3	
4	
5	
6	
7	
8	
9	
10	
11	

STRETCH COMMENTS

CARDIO

TIME/DISTANCE	COMMENTS

HOW DO YOU FEEL

BEFORE THE SESSION

AFTER THE SESSION

comments

WEEKLY SUMMARY   DATE

GOALS MET

GOALS EXCEEDED

NEXT WEEK

STRETCHING NOTES

CARDIO NOTES

DIETARY NOTES

WEEK 7

OBJECTIVES

DATE

MONDAY

STRETCHES

1	
2	
3	
4	
5	
6	
7	
8	
9	
10	
11	

STRETCH COMMENTS

CARDIO

TIME/DISTANCE	COMMENTS

HOW DO YOU FEEL

BEFORE THE SESSION

AFTER THE SESSION

TUESDAY

STRETCHES

1	
2	
3	
4	
5	
6	
7	
8	
9	
10	
11	

STRETCH COMMENTS

CARDIO

TIME/DISTANCE	COMMENTS

HOW DO YOU FEEL

BEFORE THE SESSION

AFTER THE SESSION

WEDNESDAY

STRETCHES

1	
2	
3	
4	
5	
6	
7	
8	
9	
10	
11	

STRETCH COMMENTS

CARDIO

TIME/DISTANCE	COMMENTS

HOW DO YOU FEEL

BEFORE THE SESSION

AFTER THE SESSION

THURSDAY

STRETCHES

1	
2	
3	
4	
5	
6	
7	
8	
9	
10	
11	

STRETCH COMMENTS

CARDIO

TIME/DISTANCE	COMMENTS

HOW DO YOU FEEL

BEFORE THE SESSION

AFTER THE SESSION

diet notes

Looking around you to see people running faster than you, lifting heavier weights than you, or tearing past you in the pool can be very demotivating. Try not to let what you cannot do interfere with what you can presently do.

take a break

If you often feel tired or sore after training, take a break. You can either rest up for a week, or cut down on the length and intensity of your workout. Your body is telling you that it needs to recover. You'll soon feel reenergized.

diet notes

FRIDAY

STRETCHES

1	
2	
3	
4	
5	
6	
7	
8	
9	
10	
11	

STRETCH COMMENTS

CARDIO

TIME/DISTANCE	COMMENTS

HOW DO YOU FEEL

BEFORE THE SESSION

AFTER THE SESSION

SATURDAY

STRETCHES

1	
2	
3	
4	
5	
6	
7	
8	
9	
10	
11	

STRETCH COMMENTS

CARDIO

TIME/DISTANCE	COMMENTS

HOW DO YOU FEEL

BEFORE THE SESSION

AFTER THE SESSION

SUNDAY

STRETCHES

1	
2	
3	
4	
5	
6	
7	
8	
9	
10	
11	

STRETCH COMMENTS

CARDIO

TIME/DISTANCE	COMMENTS

HOW DO YOU FEEL

BEFORE THE SESSION

AFTER THE SESSION

comments

WEEKLY SUMMARY   DATE

GOALS MET

GOALS EXCEEDED

NEXT WEEK

STRETCHING NOTES

CARDIO NOTES

DIETARY NOTES

WEEK 8

DATE

OBJECTIVES

MONDAY

STRETCHES

1	
2	
3	
4	
5	
6	
7	
8	
9	
10	
11	

STRETCH COMMENTS

CARDIO

TIME/DISTANCE	COMMENTS

HOW DO YOU FEEL

BEFORE THE SESSION

AFTER THE SESSION

TUESDAY

STRETCHES

1	
2	
3	
4	
5	
6	
7	
8	
9	
10	
11	

STRETCH COMMENTS

CARDIO

TIME/DISTANCE	COMMENTS

HOW DO YOU FEEL

BEFORE THE SESSION

AFTER THE SESSION

WEDNESDAY

STRETCHES

1	
2	
3	
4	
5	
6	
7	
8	
9	
10	
11	

STRETCH COMMENTS

CARDIO

TIME/DISTANCE	COMMENTS

HOW DO YOU FEEL

BEFORE THE SESSION

AFTER THE SESSION

THURSDAY

STRETCHES

1	
2	
3	
4	
5	
6	
7	
8	
9	
10	
11	

STRETCH COMMENTS

CARDIO

TIME/DISTANCE	COMMENTS

HOW DO YOU FEEL

BEFORE THE SESSION

AFTER THE SESSION

diet notes

Sport should always be fun. If it is not, you will quickly become demoralized and defeated by the very thing that can help bring you health and happiness. Always look out for ways of bringing some joy to your play.

all stitched up

Stitches are that annoying sharp pain below your ribs and are caused by cramping in the stomach wall. To cure them, simply stop and touch your toes a few times or breathe deeply from your stomach until the cramp passes.

diet notes

FRIDAY

STRETCHES	
1	
2	
3	
4	
5	
6	
7	
8	
9	
10	
11	

STRETCH COMMENTS

CARDIO

TIME/DISTANCE	COMMENTS

HOW DO YOU FEEL

BEFORE THE SESSION

AFTER THE SESSION

SATURDAY

STRETCHES	
1	
2	
3	
4	
5	
6	
7	
8	
9	
10	
11	

STRETCH COMMENTS

CARDIO

TIME/DISTANCE	COMMENTS

HOW DO YOU FEEL

BEFORE THE SESSION

AFTER THE SESSION